Our Voices:

First-Person Accounts of Schizophrenia

*A collection of personal experiences of
people with schizophrenia in a
small community in central North Carolina.*

Edited by

Colette Corr
Michael Dunne
Manisha Kapil
Claudia Moon
Pickens Miller

iUniverse, Inc.
New York   Bloomington

Our Voices: First-Person Accounts of Schizophrenia

iUniverse books may be ordered through booksellers or by contacting:

iUniverse
1663 Liberty Drive
Bloomington, IN 47403
www.iuniverse.com
1-800-Authors (1-800-288-4677)

ISBN: 978-1-4401-1039-9 (pbk)
ISBN: 978-1-4401-1040-5 (ebk)

Printed in the United States of America

iUniverse rev. date: 12/09/2008

This book was created by patient-authors from the Schizophrenia Treatment and Evaluation Program, Department of Psychiatry.

Acknowledgments

The publication of *Our Voices* was made possible by a generous gift to the Schizophrenia Treatment and Evaluation Program, Department of Psychiatry, School of Medicine, University of North Carolina at Chapel Hill. Cover art by Colette Corr. Cover design by Shawn Bauguess and Jen Yuson.

Saying No to the Voices

– Angela Stroud

Voices came
Voices went
Scary voices
Weird voices
Loud voices
Still small voices.

The voices tell me I'm special—
I'm somebody.

The voices tell me through the TV to listen.
I have a special message for you.

The voices came
The voices go, the voices stay
They are slow
They are not my voices
But their voices –

I say No!

Contents

A basic description of the symptoms of schizophrenia:

Positive Symptoms:

Hallucinations or false perceptions—some people hear things that other people don't hear, or see things other people don't see. Some people even feel and smell things that others don't. Hallucinations may come from the same part of our brain that creates dreams, and some people describe it as feeling like they are dreaming, even when they are awake.

Delusions, or false beliefs—some people believe things that can't possibly be true, or for which they don't have any evidence. In some cases, they will continue to believe these things even in the face of evidence that they are wrong.

Negative Symptoms:

Disorganized or catatonic behavior—some people engage in strange behaviors that seem to have no purpose to other people. Sometimes they become catatonic and do very little, not even moving their bodies unless directed to. (This is very rare.)

Lack of motivation and happiness—some people find they can no longer get started doing things, or that they no longer feel joy and happiness doing things they used to like. Some people say they feel flat, and they may get a flat tone to their voice.

Social withdrawal—some people find it very difficult to be social and become anxious around other people. This may result in a loss of school time or work.

Cognitive Symptoms:

Cognitive problems—some people experience difficulty thinking, focusing, remembering, and learning. Sometimes they find it's difficult to think abstractly, and they start to think of things in a very concrete way.

People who have schizophrenia may have some or all of these symptoms. Schizophrenia can look very different in different people.

How We Wrote the Book

Our Voices: First-Person Accounts of Schizophrenia is the first book of its type. There are similar books on schizophrenia, one where patient-authors ask the questions and share their first episodes. Our book is different in that it was designed to emphasize that schizophrenia is a lifelong illness with long-term and daily challenges, not isolating the focus on initial episodes. The market also has books with a similar format to ours: some interview and ask questions to experts, and some attempt to record or analyze answers from the popular mainstream. It should be pointed out that the subject matter of the interviews in these books varies greatly from ours.

The commitment and long process of writing and editing our own book became a reality when Jenny Edwards, one of the social workers from the UNC STEP Clinic (the University of North Carolina Schizophrenia Treatment and Evaluation Program) recognized the potential of one of many ideas that were proposed to her. It is so incredible that she would choose an idea, and have the vision, faith and confidence in us that we would make it happen! Her colleague Bebe Smith, Director of Outpatient Services at the STEP Clinic (who has worked in publishing), put the process in motion. Technically, Bebe and Jenny were just advisors for our book project, but we relied greatly on them, much more than they would have liked.

Our team of author-editors consisted of five individuals, each with some form of schizophrenia, who have weathered the worst part of their illness, have put their lives back together, and have really started to succeed in life again. Our author-editing team consists of talented writers, some accomplished, some truly solid. Because of all the unique battles we have triumphed over, we started this book project to share our personal perspectives with the world. Our goal is to develop understanding in our readers that schizophrenia is a life-long illness, as well as an understanding of shared perceptions, experiences, and challenges people with schizophrenia face in daily living and throughout the course of their illness.

After assembling the team, right away we started compiling questions for the pilot questionnaire. Each team member submitted a minimum of 10 questions. We even had a "question hog" who submitted over ninety, further complicating the process. We were seeking appropriate questions on a balance of issues pertaining to all areas relevant to the illness and lifestyle choices. Together we rewrote, rephrased, eliminated, and selected questions to evoke significant short answers. After the answers to 10 pilot questionnaires, including our own, were recorded and analyzed, we went through the process again.

The final questionnaire was in two parts, and at the end of each part, we gave the patient-authors an opportunity to write more free-form comments, which we later dubbed "elaborations."

Not every question applied to every patient-author. We also explained to them that they didn't have to answer every question to participate. To obtain honest and open answers, we chose to identify each answer from the patient-authors by a fake first name, followed by their real age. The patient-authors had a lot of fun choosing their own fake first names.

The vast majority reported they had schizoaffective disorder, some were unaware of their clinical disorder, and some declined to say. Being patients ourselves, we had no way of verifying the professional diagnosis of these patient-authors. Our final sample actually turned out to be very diverse, even though it probably didn't mirror an exact statistical model of the community. The average age was 42. We selected a final total of 20 answers – from 10 women and 10 men – to the questionnaires.

We recruited patient-authors from our friends, patients of our social work advisors, the hospital waiting room, two different clubhouses, the STEP art gallery reception, and organizations including NAMI and Schizophrenics Anonymous.

Our "book committee" officially met about once a month at the hospital to report on our progress and make pertinent decisions. We had many heated discussions, one of which resolved not to use the term "consumer," unless the patient-author made reference to it. Our discussions were so thorough that we usually came to agreements without voting.

To delve deeper into the motivation and individual psyches of people with mental illness, we included a poem in each chapter. We had enormous interest from people wanting their poetry to be published. The criteria for the poetry submitted were different than for the questionnaire. The poets were only required to have some form of mental illness. We concluded that most people with schizophrenia could compare and other readers relate to poetry about all types of mental illness, whether the poems were about depression, medication, mood disorders, or other aspects of mental illness.

Our author-editor team decided against preparing scientific chapters usually contained in books similar to ours. We decided it would be doing a disservice to the reader to oversimplify or summarize scientific explanations and findings of brain chemistry or give a condensed primer of medications and therapies. We recommend that the reader consult a number of good, updated and specialized books currently available on the market. In most chapters we have, however, provided some facts relevant to the subject of that chapter in an effort to give some background necessary to understand the questions and answers. The sources are documented in the back of the book. If you are interested in good informational websites and books, please consult the bibliography, but also keep in mind that many more excellent resources are out there.

This is a serious subject with intensely probing questions. After we studied the answers, we realized that there was not only levity in the answers but some were downright humorous. After reading this book, no one can say that people with schizophrenia don't have a sense of humor.

To read this book, you not only need to employ a similar sense of humor but an open mind. Basically, this is a book of opinions and perspectives. It entails varied perceptions and personal solutions to the challenges we face. To attempt to understand the answers at all, you need to attempt not to judge or discern.

The opinions expressed in this book are extremely varied and personal. Some are consenting, some dissenting, some rational, and some irrational. (Of course, some irrationality can be expected when dealing with people with schizophrenia.) We are not issuing the standard disclaimer about not being responsible for the opinions of others. Neither are we going to apologize for the opinions of others. We have assembled these questions and are printing them exactly as the patient-authors wrote and expressed them. Even our team members do not always agree with each other's opinions.

This book doesn't need to be read in one sitting. It does not need to be read in sequence. You may pick it up and choose any chapter. You may even single out and follow the answers of one or two people throughout the book. To digest the full meaning of the poems, you can easily read them by themselves. The elaborations, however, become more meaningful if you are acquainted with some of the answers concerning the background of the patient-author who is writing them. The facts interspersed in the chapters are popular knowledge you may already be acquainted with. Then again, you may be surprised by them.

We took the opportunity at the end of the process for each of us on the committee to have our individual voices heard. We each expressed our hopes for a brighter future for people with mental illness.

For individuals with schizophrenia—here's your chance to compare! For mental health care professionals, not only can you attempt to relate to us better—you may read what the patient-authors really think about you. (Yes, we are talking about you—see how that feels!) For the families of individuals with schizophrenia—if you seek to understand us, we're easier to live with! And for the readers who are just interested—we will rid you of stigma for good. And for us, *Our Voices* have been heard in reality and will have made a difference.

Illness and Recovery

A man who is "of sound mind" is one who keeps the inner madness under lock and key.

– Paul Valery

Manic Depression

— *Danny Green*

Insane sorrow wells
up the confines
of pain-racked being
empty of all
save nothing you feel.

Feeble edges cut
down the life-stream
of joy-filled ranting
they damn the laugh
and squelch the squeal of love.

Arid kerchiefs dry
up the teardrops
of white-stained wailing
but what is left?
A mad sneer of shame.

What is your diagnosis? Do you think it is accurate? Why or why not?

Jade, 43: Schizoaffective and PTSD. Yes. I have severe mood swings (affective); I see and hear things (schizo); I have a trauma history (PTSD).

Socrates, 43: My diagnosis is schizoaffective disorder. Originally it was bipolar disorder, but was changed. I believe it is accurate.

Adam, 28: Undetermined type schizophrenia. Yes, the doctors determined delusions and hallucinations, among others.

Danny Green, 46: Schizoaffective disorder. Psychiatric diagnoses are all highly imprecise and shall remain so until we discover underlying causes.

Brunhilda, 44: My diagnosis is schizoaffective disorder. I don't like the name, but it includes all of my major symptoms.

Zelda, 48: Chronic paranoid schizophrenia. No. Because the diagnosis came in a court setting and not a doctor's office.

Will, 38: Schizoaffective, bipolar type. I believe it is accurate because in the past I have had trouble with significant mood swings, delusional thinking, and some hallucinations.

> In Greek, "schiz" or "schizo" means "split." Thus, schizophrenia means split from reality, which an individual undergoing a psychotic episode experiences. It does not mean an individual has a "split" or multiple personality (en.wikipedia.org/wiki/Schizophrenia).

Jane, 53: My diagnosis is schizoaffective disorder. I think it is accurate because my doctors have been able to find some medicines that did help me, and because I thought I might have schizophrenia, even in childhood.

Barnaby, 23: Schizoaffective disorder. I do think it's accurate; I have symptoms I know to be psychotic that get worse when I'm down or depressed.

Harriet, 43: Borderline personality disorder and schizoaffective. Yes, I have been in treatment with two psychiatrists for a span of almost 30 years, and have received help for these diagnoses.

Ozzie, 46: Paranoid schizophrenia.

Diagnosing schizophrenia is done through interview and observation. There are no blood tests or brain scans that can tell us a person has schizophrenia. A doctor may request tests to rule out underlying causes, but schizophrenia does not show up on imaging tests or other physical exams.

Larry, 46: I try to not pay much attention to a diagnosis. I try to focus on living with my illness outside of a diagnosis.

Jill, 27: Schizoaffective is accurate because I have psychotic symptoms while not depressed or manic.

Aileen, 54: Paranoid schizophrenia. Yes, my symptoms fit the diagnosis.

Black Madonna, 36: Schizoaffective disorder. No! I believe I have been misdiagnosed. I believe I suffer from some depression only. I have "Graves Disease." I had a medical treatment on my thyroid. I believe I suffer from depression because my thyroid is out of order.

Christen, 44: My diagnosis is schizoaffective disorder. I think it is accurate because it includes all my symptoms.

Brian, 43: Schizoaffective disorder. Yes, I think it is accurate. It makes sense to me because I have both psychosis and depression.

Jay, 56: Schizoaffective, post-traumatic stress disorder. I believe this diagnosis is correct because my symptoms agree with the determinations of the illness cited.

Rachel, 44: I am schizoaffective and obsessive compulsive. I feel that these diagnoses are accurate. The schizo part of my diagnosis reflects the fact that I am sometimes not able to identify or recognize reality. The affective part reflects that there is a mood component, or moodiness, to my illness. Because I am obsessive compulsive, I tend to dwell on this moodiness or on false perceptions of reality.

Liana, 50: Schizophrenia—I don't think it's accurate because I was told I had anxiety neurosis in 1972.

How do you describe your illness?

Jade, 43: I say sometimes I get depressed, and sometimes I hear voices.

Socrates, 43: The main symptoms I deal with are anxiety, some paranoia, and some obsessive thinking. I don't respond well to stress.

Adam, 28: The same as the doctor.

Danny Green, 46: A physical shutdown of the central nervous system. A brain disease like any other—comparable to Parkinson's or Alzheimer's.

Brunhilda, 44: Psychotic and bipolar all at the same time, with a large amount of negative symptoms.

Zelda, 48: I don't know. I have tinnitus and sometimes it gets confused with auditory hallucinations.

Will, 38: In remission, well managed with medication and self care.

Jane, 53: Lately, I have been feeling much better than before, but I still have many qualms about doing things.

Barnaby, 23: Schizoaffective disorder is like being drawn into another world. Reality changes to suit your fears and anxieties.

> Dr. Emil Kraeplin first identified schizophrenia as a mental illness in 1887, but the illness was coined "schizophrenia" by the Swiss psychiatrist Eugene Bleuler in 1911 (en.wikipedia. org/wiki/Schizophrenia).

Harriet, 43: High anxiety, depression, and without medication, psychosis.

Ozzie, 46: I had delusions about God and life.

Larry, 46: I have limitations in my life due to thought processes.

Jill, 27: Psychosis, full blown mania, as well as hypomania and depression—which I haven't had in a while—and anxiety.

Aileen, 54: I had delusions and magical thinking, as well as physical hallucinations. I heard and hear voices, also.

Black Madonna, 36: There are periods when I feel really down and hopeless. There are times when I experience anxiety and stress a lot. When I spend lots of money, and I can stay up for days, cleaning up— my illness gives me highs and low feelings emotionally.

Christen, 44: Frustrating at times.

Brian, 43: As a biological brain disease caused by a chemical imbalance.

Jay, 56: Psychotic, depression and anxiety.

Liana, 50: Depressing.

What was it like to discover you had a mental illness? How did you come to that understanding? What did it mean to you?

Jade, 43: I guess I always knew. I had my first hallucination when I was 8. It was a relief to finally get some treatment. And the diagnosis helped put a name on that which had been destroying my life for years. With an identifiable name I could begin to address it and begin to heal.

Socrates, 43: My first reaction to my illness was deep depression. I thought of taking my life, but I feared God too much to do so. I wasn't sure suicide would end my suffering. Coming to grips with my illness took time. I knew that something was wrong, but I thought that God would heal me, which led to noncompliance with medication. Eventually I realized that though God would heal me to a large extent, emotionally and psychologically, the physical aspect of my illness would persist.

> Although we don't know all the risk factors of schizophrenia, theories about risk factors include genetics, unbalanced brain chemistry, possible viral infections, and immune disorders. When a genetic predisposition exists, environmental factors also can play a role in developing the illness (Meuser and Gingrich 5).

Adam, 28: Relief. That there was a reason. A doctor understood. Some resolution.

Danny Green, 46: Terrifying. I knew it years before I was diagnosed. I could sense the onslaught of the annihilation of purpose. My brain had shut down.

Brunhilda, 44: I became extremely confused, depressed, and suicidal when I realized I was psychotic. I didn't understand if I should tell someone or where to go for help. I just slept all the time. When I did go for help, they hospitalized me right away. The hospital gave me hope, through educating me about my illness.

Zelda, 48: It stinks. I was in a state of rage. The diagnosing physician said that I would hate her for the diagnosis. I was 45. I was trapped.

Individuals with mental illness often delay seeking treatment for up to 10 years, and this delay increases "the likeliness of disability and negative social outcomes." Delaying treatment also results in greater numbers of symptoms and frequency of episodes (Uninsured and Costs 8).

Will, 38: Very disturbing, unsettling, disorienting. My path in life was disrupted for quite some time. At the beginning, insight was somewhat poor, and this affected my recovery.

Jane, 53: I was still a child when I thought I might have schizophrenia. When I was in my forties, I was told that I could have an illness that might last the rest of my life. I found it depressing to be told that. I believe that God can heal me if he wants.

Barnaby, 23: Looking back, I had my first full-blown psychotic symptoms when I was 18. After putting my hand through a window, I was sent to an inpatient psych ward where I learned of my illness. It meant that I couldn't function in certain respects. It meant that I'd lost something of myself. I felt lame.

Harriet, 43: I was 15 at the onset. I did not understand it. I knew I was different from other people. I could not accept myself.

Ozzie, 46: Thirty-five years old. I felt like everybody was out to get me.

Larry, 46: Scary. I was hospitalized at 19. It meant having to learn to live my life differently than I was accustomed to.

Jill, 27: I've had mental illness since I was quite young. Didn't get diagnosed until I was 16. I was relieved. It meant I could finally get the help I deserved.

Aileen, 54: It was devastating, and a relief at the same time. I came to the understanding over a period of time after I was first hospitalized. I was 42 years old. It meant the delusions stopped (I didn't miss them), and the magical thinking (which I missed).

Black Madonna, 36: It was heartbreaking. I was embarrassed. When I was 11 years old I was sad a lot and very introverted and shy. I didn't understand. I had no clue about mental illness—it scared me being so young.

Christen, 44: I thought the world was coming to an end. When I got better, I understood I had a mental illness. I was 25 years old then.

Brian, 43: It was very painful. I did not understand it until I found myself in a state hospital. I was 21 years old. At the time it felt to me like my life was hopeless and I had no future.

Jay, 56: In a way, good, for there was an explanation for what I was experiencing. I came to this understanding by way of acceptance of mental health workers. I had a mental illness; next, resolve it.

Rachel, 44: I had my first break with reality when I was 22. When I was 25 I had my second break. The first time I was very paranoid and felt universally hated. The second time, I was obsessed with death and dying and did not feel safe from attack by others. I felt like I was the only one who knew what was really going on.

Liana, 50: I felt betrayed—people would say, "That's your schizophrenia." I was 21. It meant that people were no longer compassionate.

What would you say to someone who has just found out they have a major mental illness?

Jade, 43: Get all the information you can. Be your own best advocate. There is no "they." It is a cooperative effort with the doctors to help heal you.

Schizophrenia usually strikes men in their late teens and early twenties, and women later, in their twenties and thirties (schizophrenia.com/szfacts.htm).

Socrates, 43: The first thing I would tell someone who was diagnosed with mental illness is that there is hope. Just because you may feel miserable now doesn't mean you will always feel this way.

Adam, 28: Learn. Accept it. Learn to manage it. Things could definitely get better.

Danny Green, 46: There is hope.

Brunhilda, 44: I would explain to them that their illness is a chemical imbalance. Also, that whether or not there is a drug to alleviate their symptoms, there will be one in the future. I would want them to know that the psychiatrists are only gambling on which medications will help. They should keep trying, and that it is a very long process.

Zelda, 48: It stinks. Make sure you know the doctor very well. Do not meet them in court.

The incidence of schizophrenia is 1% worldwide, and in the U.S. at least 40% are not receiving treatment (www.schizophrenia.com/szfacts.htm).

Will, 38: You are not the first, you are not alone, and you are not to blame. However, should you accept this challenge, diagnosis, and label in life, your wellness and life progress are ultimately your responsibility.

Jane, 53: I would say, "I'm sorry that this has happened to you," very gently.

Barnaby, 23: I'd say, "Join the club." I've found that communities of people with mental illness often have stronger ties than communities without mental illness. I met my best friend in a psych ward.

Harriet, 43: Have compassion for yourself. Trust your doctors—don't hold back. Have hope. Trust in your higher power.

Ozzie, 46: Get help.

Larry, 46: Listen to what others are trying to say to you.

Jill, 27: There is hope.

Aileen, 54: Hang in there. It gets easier. Find friends and outside interests.

Black Madonna, 36: I would tell them to learn all they can about their illness – get into a support group. And join Club Nova* – where I attend. It's a place for people who have something in common with each other. (*Editors' note: Club Nova is the local club house. It follows the Fountain House model and has national accreditation.)

Christen, 44: I would say to someone who has just found out they have a mental illness to be patient with yourself and pray a lot.

Brian, 43: I would say, "Hang in there and things really can get better in time." Find a medication that works well for you and find a program for support or therapy.

Jay, 56: Try and accept yourself having the condition. Most illnesses are treatable and can be managed.

Rachel, 44: Find a knowledgeable, experienced and empathetic psychiatrist. Don't be afraid to try the medicines he or she prescribes. If a medicine isn't working, ask your psychiatrist to prescribe something else. The benefits of the right drug for you greatly outweigh the problems with side effects. You will actually find great emotional relief when you are on that medicine, and most of the difficulties you have been facing will improve.

Liana, 50: Tell that person there is hope.

What, for you, is the most difficult aspect of your illness?

Jade, 43: The dread that overcomes me right before I begin hallucinating.

Socrates, 43: The most difficult aspect of my illness is probably dealing with the emotion of fear, and with prejudice and misjudgment of others. Because I have this illness, many people believe that I am somehow weak and incapable. But those who know me well, know that I am neither.

Adam, 28: Its persistence and its consistency.

Danny Green, 46: Gaps in gainful employment.

Brunhilda, 44: Being bipolar is the greatest hindrance for me. I am highly functioning when I suffer delusions or hallucinations. However, it is the cycling from mania to depression that keeps me from functioning effectively.

Zelda, 48: Taking medications and always being fatigued. Being strapped by the medication. You see, I don't believe that I am ill, but I can't go off the medication to find out.

Will, 38: For some years, it was my stagnation in life, lack of motivation, apathy and morning depression.

Jane, 53: The most difficult aspect of my illness has been that the doctors said that if God did heal me, they would find it very difficult to tell, which makes me, in effect, a prisoner of the medical establishment, with medicines, the side effects of which are not easy to tolerate.

Barnaby, 23: The negative symptoms. It's hard to get back what you've lost, and the medication seems to help the positive symptoms more quickly than the negative ones. Positive symptoms make your life crazy; the negative ones take your life away.

Harriet, 43: Even today—feeling like I am losing control of my mind, when tired and anxious.

Ozzie, 46: Having to take medicine every day.

Larry, 46: My mind is "playing tricks on me."

Jill, 27: It's a life-long process with many challenges and frequent medication changes.

Aileen, 54: Having to regulate my life around my disorder.

Black Madonna, 36: Sleeping a lot—feeling like you want to pass on before your time—feelings of happiness—mania—feeling high—not getting enough sleep at night. Staying up for three or four days at a time.

Christen, 44: Getting through the panic and anxiety.

Brian, 43: Depression and low self-esteem.

Jay, 56: The limits it places on my life.

Rachel, 44: It frustrates me that as a side effect of my medicine, my thoughts are slowed down and I cannot think intellectually as efficiently and capably as I used to (before medicine).

Liana, 50: Feeling uncovered.

If you have ever been suicidal, can you tell us about that? What has helped you through those tough times?

Jade, 43: If I am getting command hallucinations to kill myself, I need outside help—extra doctor's appointments, staying with my family. If it gets really bad, I go to the hospital.

Socrates, 43: I have had suicidal thoughts, but I have never acted on them because I feared what God might do to me if I gave up. At my lowest moment, I did eventually give up and prayed for death, but God sustained me.

Adam, 28: I have been suicidal—there was always some inkling that things would improve. Hope.

Danny Green, 46: When I have been, what helped was time itself.

Brunhilda, 44: The problem with being suicidal and telling a mental healthcare professional is that they almost always hospitalize you. I feel more depressed people would seek their help if there wasn't this threat. What helps me through these tough times is to think about my boyfriend and family, and convince myself they need me.

Zelda, 48: After the diagnosis, who wouldn't be? My mother and my therapist.

Will, 38: I was fundamentally suicidal and obsessed with death for about 15 years—all my thoughts gravitated to darkness and despair. Ultimately my commitment to myself and my life prevailed.

Jane, 53: When I was faintly suicidal, I thought I had done something unforgivable. For a long time, I was not aware that the Lord could forgive me; but finally, He got the message through that He did. Meanwhile, I had several hospital stays and the comforts of home to get me through the difficult times. It helped that people paid attention to me and tried to help me. I also had a prayer partner who helped me by saying that she was convinced I hadn't committed an unforgivable sin and that the Lord was going to help me believe that I had not. I think that prayers helped me through the hard times very much.

Barnaby, 23: I have been suicidal, and I can tell you that when you are in that mindset, thinking about ending your life is kind of a release. That's why I kept thinking about it but putting it off. Thinking that you only have a few days left makes those days stress-free and almost fun because nothing matters, and then you don't feel pressed to actually do it. What got me through? Now that I believe in God, I would never attempt it again, but at the time, I couldn't fully pull myself away from people. I couldn't stand the idea of never seeing them again.

Harriet, 43: I have had suicidal thoughts but never acted on them. I am not afraid to ask for help—that has helped me.

Larry, 46: Yes, I wanted the pain and discomfort to end. Hospitalizations to a certain point.

Jill, 27: I was in my teens. I felt like the world was ending, and it was my fault, and if I died, then the world would be better place. What helped me was family support.

Aileen, 54: I have thought about suicide during several periods over the past 12 years. Knowing I have children and that they need me got me through these times.

Black Madonna, 36: No! I've only prayed that God would take me to heaven when I have had really tough times—I have never wanted to kill myself. But I have lied to the doctor about it, just to get in the hospital so I could get some sleep.

Christen, 44: My husband has always been there when I was suicidal. A few times he has stopped me.

Brian, 43: Yes. I have been suicidal in the past. It always helped me to know that I could go to the hospital where I would be safe. Also, finding a good medication that worked very well for me may have actually saved my life.

Suicide is a major cause of premature death in people with schizophrenia (Torrey 311). The suicide rate among people with schizophrenia is many times that in the general population. About 40% of people with schizophrenia attempt suicide, although most attempt it within the first 10 years of onset (www.schizophrenia.com/family/FAQgen.htm#suicide).

Jay, 56: I have been suicidal several times. Hospitalization has helped, as well as having a stable support system, i.e., a place to live, people to talk to.

Rachel, 44: I have been suicidal several times in my life. Almost always it is caused by my perception of being dismissed or mistreated by others. My faith in God has sustained me, the knowledge that Jesus was misunderstood and mistreated helps. Also, a passage that I read from a book about near-death experiences concluded that if one could not resolve one's problems in this life, he or she certainly would not be able to resolve them in the next life.

Liana, 50: I scratched my wrists and took an overdose in 1976. I lost weight a year later and felt in a sense, "self-actualized."

If you have or have had hallucinations or delusions, can you describe them?

Jade, 43: Bodies. The military coming to kill everybody. Dead people in the clouds speaking a special language to me.

> **Paranoid delusions** are beliefs that people want to harm you.
> **Delusions of reference** are beliefs that things in your environment are directly related to you (like special communications from the TV or radio).
> **Somatic delusions** are incorrect beliefs about your body.
> **Delusions of grandeur** are beliefs that you are very important or have special abilities (Miller and Mason 38).

Socrates, 43: I have had both auditory and visual hallucinations, as those in the profession would call them, but I call them inner locutions and visions. All of these have been spiritual in nature. One of them involved seeing a vision of a mountain, and I was traveling up the mountain to see God.

Adam, 28: Scary. Maybe from God. Wonderful, awful, confused sometimes.

Brunhilda, 44: Hallucinations may sound exactly like certain people you know. However, sometimes the voices are from fictitious people in my head. Delusions get more complicated and complex the longer they go on. They are only easier to dispel when they are simple and have first begun. Apparently they are reinforced with time.

Zelda, 48: In 2001, I tried to move the family from Raleigh to Washington, DC. As we had resided in France for 20 years, this hallucination could have been interpreted as a pragmatic thing to do.

Will, 38: Auditory and visual hallucinations, not to any really significant degree. Grandiose and delusional thinking was the real enemy for quite some time.

Jane, 53: Sometimes I have imagined, or thought that I had seen, weird shapes.

Barnaby, 23: Wow. I've had many delusions. I've thought everything from being a rock star followed around by invisible cameras to having old high school friends that I couldn't see follow me around. I used to have conversations with crickets and birds (actually, I still do—I know it's weird), and at one point, I thought the damned were in my backyard. Perhaps one of the most intrusive delusions was that everyone in the world was constantly watching me on a giant TV screen. As far as hallucinations go, I hear demons. I do think they're real; that is, the demons are not a delusion.

Harriet, 43: Off medication at age 25 I worked in a restaurant. I believed that my manager, who was married to the head waitress, was going to leave her and marry me. I called my doctor the night I thought he was going to marry me, and he said, "Take 50 mg of Mellaril and another 50 mg and another 50 mg." He has treated me for 24 years, and I have never had to be hospitalized.

Ozzie, 46: Yes, I had delusions about God and different life systems that could exist; delusions about creation.

> While auditory hallucinations are the most common, people can hallucinate in any of the five senses (Miller and Mason 38).

Larry, 46: Voices that you try to understand and figure out. Seeing things that are not there, regardless of how real they seem.

Jill, 27: Television talking to me, people I know appearing on TV, beliefs that my insides were rotting out, etc.

Aileen, 54: I have had physical hallucinations that feel like I am being stabbed. My delusions were about making positive changes in the world when "in control" and doing damage in the world when out of control.

Black Madonna, 36: Yes! I have had hallucinations where I saw and heard something or someone that wasn't really there.

Christen, 44: One time I thought my arm was on fire and people were reading my mind. One time when my husband was driving fast, I thought I was going to be splattered all over the road. All these things were very real to me.

Brian, 43: Yes, I have had delusions of persecution where I thought that people were conspiring against me. I was very paranoid and frightened.

Jay, 56: I've experienced auditory and visual hallucinations as well as delusions. Typically they've been about mental health workers, both audio and visual. The delusions have been like I was living out some kind of spy novel.

Liana, 50: I saw a face in a tree outside my window in September of 1975.

How has your life changed because of your mental illness?

Jade, 43: I lost my marriage, my career, my hope for having children.

Socrates, 43: I have had to face the realization that my chosen profession (teaching) is too stressful for me and that I must limit my stress to function well.

Adam, 28: Gotten better. Away from and over the exacerbating pressures of day-to-day strain.

Danny Green, 46: No education, no career.

Brunhilda, 44: I've been mentally ill so long, it's my way of life. There is no way I can speculate how my life would be different after 25 years!

> Schizophrenia is a lifelong illness with an episodic course, whose symptoms vary in intensity at different times. During episodes chronic symptoms worsen and those in remission may reappear, at times requiring hospitalization (Mueser and Gingrich 13).

Zelda, 48: I get patronized by professionals.

Will, 38: For the better. I have used my experience with SPMI to improve myself as a person. I came to a better understanding of myself and others, my life, my spirit, my God.

Jane, 53: It is much harder than it was to get a job, let alone meaningful work. My family seems to be trying to decide how to deal with me as I age. Medicaid has been tremendously helpful.

Barnaby, 23: Because of my illness, I have lost friends; my sense of silliness has been covered by worries. I had to withdraw from college, and I feel I am not as capable as before. I've lost something of myself.

Harriet, 43: My life is good. I am married to a man who is a paranoid schizophrenic. We cherish each other and have great compassion for each other.

Ozzie, 46: I think it was for the better. I used to work as a construction inspector and it was hard on my body. Now I get disability and work part-time. I have a lot more free time.

There is no cure for schizophrenia, but it can be effectively treated with medication and therapy.

Jill, 27: I have understood myself better. And maybe the way others perceive me, the way I am is not my fault.

Aileen, 54: I struggle to be creative. I am an artist. I struggle with my sex life. I worry a lot. I struggle with side effects of my meds.

Black Madonna, 36: My life has changed a great deal. I used to be a child care teacher for nine years. I used to hold a job full time. I miss working full time. Financially it has been a struggle to make ends meet. I used to help my husband bring home the bacon, but now I'm on SSDI, and my bills are behind.

Christen, 44: I am not capable of doing things like I used to do. I can't hold down a job or cook like I used to do. I can only concentrate on one thing at a time.

Brian, 43: Yes. I think my life has changed a great deal. Both in bad ways and in some good ways.

Jay, 56: Yes, significantly.

Rachel, 44: Before mental illness, I was an overachiever. After mental illness I am not able to work or function normally. People (strangers) see the blank look in my eyes that comes from the medication and think that I am slow instead of mentally ill.

Liana, 50: Interdependency with the other members of Club Nova. People are supportive.

What is the best thing to happen to you in terms of your recovery, and what has helped you recover?

Jade, 43: My newfound closeness with my parents. They have helped me recover.

Socrates, 43: My relationship with God has grown more intimate. He has been my greatest support and healer.

Adam, 28: Thinking more clearly and organized. Time and therapy. Taking more and better medicine.

Danny Green, 46: My time in Massachusetts. Worthy work.

Brunhilda, 44: A psychiatric resident took a special interest in me. The second year I saw him, he conducted cognitive behavioral therapy every week with me. I had been on Clozaril for almost 10 years. Surprisingly enough, I started doing very well after he reduced it by 225 mg. Now I'm on an average amount (400 mg/day) and doing great. The best thing that happened to me in terms of my recovery is living with my boyfriend. It forced me to keep standard hours, including getting a lot of sleep. This is the best way to control the bipolar aspect of my illness.

Zelda, 48: I have made some terrific friends. The STEP Clinic and my therapist.

Will, 38: It was a test of stamina, tenacity and faith. The battle is never really over. I plan to die fighting.

Jane, 53: My family is convinced that being on my current medication, Zyprexa, has helped me tremendously. It also helped me enormously to be told I was forgiven for the things I had done that bothered me. Physical activity has sometimes helped me, too.

Barnaby, 23: The best thing to happen to me in terms of my recovery is Clozaril. I've got my mind back; instead of my head reeling over delusions and filled with hallucinated voices, I have control for the most part. And now I can think about what I want to think about. I couldn't do that before. Religion has helped me recover. Even if someone didn't believe in God, I think he or she could see how believing in God could help someone who believes demons are talking to him.

Harriet, 43: I think seeing my husband get mentally sick after we were married, with no prior mental health history, helped me to accept myself and my illness.

Ozzie, 46: I haven't been ill in nine years. I think my wife had a great deal to do with my recovery.

After 20 years, of the people diagnosed with schizophrenia:
- 25% completely recover
- 25% are much improved and relatively independent
- 25% are improved but require an extensive support network
- 15% are hospitalized and unimproved
- 10% are dead (many from suicide)

After 30 years, of the people diagnosed with schizophrenia:
- 25% completely recover
- 35% are much improved and relatively independent
- 15% are improved but require an extensive support network
- 10% are hospitalized, unimproved
- 15% are dead (many from suicide)

(Torrey 106)

Larry, 46: Becoming employed in a mental health program. Trying to not make the same mistake twice.

Jill, 27: A wonderful doctor helped me discover Clozaril, which changed my life. Basically, helped me to live again.

Aileen, 54: My women's group with other women with similar disorders. I waited for years for contact like we have in group—good friendships, good social workers have helped me recover.

Black Madonna, 36: I pray. I study the holy scriptures. I put my faith in God and Jesus. I started attending Club Nova five years ago, and this is a big reason for my recovery. Being around others with mental illness. Being able to socialize with people at Club Nova.

Christen, 44: Prayer and my medicine have helped me recover. My husband is the best thing that has happened to me in terms of recovery.

Brian, 43: I started a drug called Clozapine or Clozaril around 14 years ago, and it has worked so well for me that I have not had even one hospitalization since then.

Jay, 56: Being placed on medication that helped me to control my behavior. I'm still in the process of recovering but what has also been a lot of help is having a stable place to stay and attending therapy.

Rachel, 44: The best thing about recovery is a renewed sense of peace in my life after taking medications, and improved relations with others after therapy. Therapy also helped me realize that many of my interpersonal difficulties were just as much the other person's fault as mine. I no longer felt so much shame and guilt over problem relationships.

Liana, 50: The best thing that happened to me is that I lost weight. I felt a sense of self esteem.

Elaborations...

Jade, 43: "You don't belong here, you're a KENNEDY," the girl with the teddy bear who wore 20 scarves around her head cornered me and yelled.

"It's your teeth," my mom comforted me on the pay phone in the hall that night, a line of people behind me, some to talk to a real person, some just to yell into the receiver for their allotted 10 minutes.

She was right, though, that teddy bear girl. I didn't belong here. Here people ate their feces, masturbated in public, broke a jaw when the TV channel was changed without approval.

Where did I belong?

The community hospital couldn't help me any more, my voices constantly telling me to cut off my breasts, to hang myself. My voices telling me that armed mercenaries were coming to kill us all. I was lost in delusions for days. I was too sick to be in an environment that counted on people exerting some control over their actions.

But there was that small part of me that sensed that this place was not a good place. It didn't smell good. We were all brought here in shackles.

It took a while to learn my way around, find the right people to help me, find some activity to help pass the time. But at the end of the day, we slept with one eye open. And that never changed.

Barnaby, 23: There was a time when I didn't try to ignore the voices; I'd have conversations with them. I always thought (and still think) they are demons, but I believed they could be converted to goodness and be saved. I gave the voices names that they readily used and went about my business of being nice to them, thinking they were receptive to the idea. They pretended for some time to want to be good and to try to change their ways; I went about doing what I thought I should to encourage them and get them on their way. Of course, when I realized they had no desire for salvation and that they truly were the worst creatures in all creation, I stopped talking to them. It's been a long time since then, and when I hear them now, I usually say, "Leave me alone, voices." I used to hear them constantly, but now more often than not, I don't hear them. I'd recommend to anyone who hears voices to actively ignore them—it will help in the long run.

Socrates, 44: In my darkest hour, I was homeless, thrown out on the street into a place I did not know, by a doctor who was reeling because I had won my freedom from a judge. He provided me with no medicine and no money and no way home. I had been put in a forensic unit of a psychiatric hospital because there was no room in the regular ward. Though I had committed no crime, I was housed with psychiatric criminals, and was physically and emotionally abused. I had been sent to this institution after being pulled over by the police for swerving in the road, as I hadn't slept in several days. The police had taken me to a private hospital, but because I had no insurance, they shipped me off to this public institution. But I decided that being on the street would be preferable to living in abuse. I took my chances, not knowing that I would not be provided with even medicine.

After being committed to a psychiatric ward, most, if not all, states allow you to have your case heard by a judge after a certain number of days. I had been in this ward for two weeks when a judge came in to hear my case. There was a large table flagged by an ominous group of practitioners, many of whom I had never met, but the most formidable of these was my doctor. I hesitate to call him such, for he was no healer. He was very deceptive and very spiritually powerful. My most difficult battles were with him.

Well, several practitioners made their case to keep me incarcerated. But I also had my chance. There were many lies told about my behavior, and each time a lie was spoken, I would interrupt the speaker, declaring his or her statement false. I am not sure whether the judge believed me, or that she was restricted by a law which says you must be a danger to yourself or others (and I have never displayed such behavior), but she granted me my liberty. As I have said, the doctor threw me out on the street with nothing, not even medicine.

I regressed into psychosis, coming under immense demonic attack. In two weeks' time, I found only one shelter in which I was provided a cot and a meal, but told I could stay only one day. Other than one other meal that a gracious man bought me, I did not eat for nearly two weeks, with precious little to drink as well, suffering from both starvation and dehydration. I nearly, literally froze to death. But all that physical suffering pales next to the spiritual suffering I experienced.

Doctors explain what I have experienced as psychosomatic syndrome. Psychological duress translates into perceived physical suffering.

Some of these sensations are difficult to describe and even more difficult for others, who have never had them, to understand. One night it was as if a burning stake were being thrust into my heel. Another time it was as if a heavy beam was breaking my back, and I was bent over from its weight. Still again I felt like a snake was biting into my heart. And there were worse than these, which I choose not to describe or even remember. Suffice it to say, I suffered immeasurably. Finally, one night I had taken all I could bear, and I begged God to take my life. I felt and saw the walls of Hell ascend around me, and I'm sure I experienced what it would be like to be in that place of torment. But He said, "No, you are too strong." He led me to a hill and told me He would put me to sleep and that when I awoke, things would be different. When I awoke with the sun, the demonic affliction had slackened somewhat, and I was able to go on, not because I had been strong enough to withstand my suffering, but because God had sustained me.

From that point, which I considered the nadir of my existence, God led me to a hospital, and I thought that at last I would get some help, but I was mistaken. They also shipped me off to a different state institution, and I did not imagine the snare that the devil had waiting for me. In my frail condition, he had prepared a place for me that would make even the forensic unit seem appealing. I cannot fully describe what I experienced when I first entered that state institution, but it was like stepping back into hell; it was not only a physical prison, but a spiritual one as well. The evil in the atmosphere defies my ability to describe, but it was thick with treachery, suffocating and dangerous, even perilous. The orderly who greeted me turned out to be the most evil person in the place, and even after I had recovered my sanity, my opinion of him did not change. That night, in my weakened condition, I had to fight for my soul, a fight that would continue with varying degrees of torment for an entire month, after which miraculously the doctor gave me my freedom, and I came back to Chapel Hill.

Here, I received assistance, and gradually, through a non-profit agency that works with the mentally ill, gained my independence and put my life back together.

Medication

There is no medicine like hope, no incentive so great, and no tonic so powerful as expectation of something tomorrow.

— Orison Swett Marden

Unsung Hero

—I. Kaldor

I feel the changing
Pressure tide.

I feel the sorrows slowly passing by
Its watching change
As carpets fly.

Hear the old rune of the division
Bell
Hear the old tune all too well
Watch it echo from within
Feel it saturate your fragile skin.

Take the time to watch the tides
Let it soothe your ailing mind
Hear a whisper in the dark
Hear it loud
Watch it spark.

What are your experiences with medications? Which have been helpful? Which have not?

Jade, 43: I have been on at least 15 medications. Now I am on 10 that are working. Clozaril seems to work the best.

Socrates, 43: Most medications I've taken over the years have added to my suffering, but seven years ago I started taking Zyprexa and have had few, if any, side effects from this medicine. It has helped keep me out of the hospital for seven years.

Adam, 28: Risperdal and Effexor have been helpful.

Danny Green, 46: Clozapril, Paxil, Depakote are working for me. None of 20 other tranquilizers or neuroleptics.

Brunhilda, 44: Clozaril was the first atypical antipsychotic that worked for me. The antidepressant Remeron changed my life because it effectively controlled the bipolar aspect of my illness. I've had many drug trials that were total failures. I seem to do well on "sleep a lot, eat a lot" medications.

Zelda, 48: Zyprexa gave me Zyprexa belly. Abilify has been helpful, I guess.

Will, 38: I have journeyed from Haldol to Navane/lithium and Cogentin with Klonopin, to experience with Risperdal, to many years of Zyprexa packing on the pounds, and now Abilify. All have been somewhat helpful, but psychopharmacology is not the sole or ultimate answer to wellness.

Jane, 53: Navane helped me for a long time; but finally I began to get symptoms of Parkinson's so I had to stop. Seroquel helped me a little but gave me an intolerable sensitivity to heat in the summertime. Trilafon helped a bit but while taking that, I once confused right and left; fortunately, my mother was driving and I was not! Thorazine made me so sleepy that I dreamt about sleeping. When I took Abilify, I had several strange reactions, of which I remember only the last one—one of my kneecaps seemed to dislocate, and I had trouble walking. Also when I was on Abilify, I became very hostile to God and man and had to be hospitalized. Switching to Zyprexa seems to have helped to solve that problem, too. Zyprexa seems to be helpful with my mood but seems as if it can sometimes make me a bit forgetful and makes it fiendishly hard to lose weight. Geodon did not work at all for me. I nearly had a nervous breakdown when I tried that.

Barnaby, 23: Clozaril is the best medication I have ever taken. The only antidepressant that has ever helped was Paxil; however, after taking it and stopping and taking it again, it doesn't do much any more.

Harriet, 43: Mellaril helped early on. Then Klonopin when it came out in 1990. Lamictal gave me bad side effects.

> Medication is an essential treatment for schizophrenia. Drugs do not cure, but control the symptoms of the illness; when other forms of treatment are combined with medication, the likelihood of improvement increases.

Ozzie, 46: I was on olanzapine, then they changed it to perphenazine, due to the costs. I haven't been ill in nine years.

Larry, 46: A long, drawn-out process of learning to comply. Clozaril and lithium.

Jill, 27: I have been on about all the atypical antipsychotics. None seemed to work, and we were giving up hope until we discovered Clozaril, which helped a lot. Lamictal also helped with my moods, where Depakote did not.

Aileen, 54: Medications cause side effects. Abilify in combination with a little Haldol has worked for me. Seroquel doesn't work. Risperdal deadened me. Ziprasadone made me anxious. Zyprexa caused me to gain a lot of weight.

Black Madonna, 36: I have been on about 20 different meds over a 15-year period. Depakote has been the worst for me, it made me gain 40 pounds, or more.

Christen, 44: I have been on so many it's hard to keep track. I remember really disliking lithium, Haldol and Depakote. I like Abilify.

Brian, 43: I take a drug called Clozaril which works very well for me. Drugs that have not worked well for me include Haldol, Prolixin, and some antidepressants.

Jay, 56: I've been on numerous medications. All have helped to some degree. Currently I am taking clozapine, which has helped me control my behavior.

Rachel, 44: I am on Haldol and Seroquel. I tried several antidepressants and Risperdal without success. Risperdal was totally ineffective for me—although I know several people who have been helped by it. The antidepressants caused insomnia, which was intolerable to me.

Liana, 50: Restlessness—Empirin codeine #3 was used for menstrual cramps and that was helpful. Also, a shot and Cogentin for restlessness.

How many psychotropic drugs are you on at present? Estimate how many medications you have tried since you developed mental illness. Which ones were acceptable? Which ones were not?

Jade, 43: I take 10 medications. I have probably tried over 20 medications. The ones that made me dizzy and faint were not acceptable.

Socrates, 43: I am on two psychotropic drugs right now: Zyprexa and Zoloft. I have tried at least nine different psychotropic drugs. Haldol,

Thorazine, Mellaril, Risperdal, lithium, Prolixin, and Navane were all unacceptable. The two I am on now work well.

Adam, 28: Two now, seven in the past. All worked to some degree.

Danny Green, 46: No one asked me whether they made ME feel better. Three are currently working, dozens have failed. I felt as if I were a gazelle on the show "Wild Kingdom."

Brunhilda, 44: I'm on two antipsychotics and one antidepressant. I've tried at least seven antipsychotics and 10 or more antidepressants and/or mood elevators. Most of these failed, but for years I got by staying on medications that were only acceptable.

Zelda, 48: One. A dozen. Zyprexa is unacceptable.

Will, 38: Depakote, Zoloft and Abilify. Zyprexa nearly devastated my physical health and hammered my self-image. I am still losing weight and recovering.

Jane, 53: I am on one medication taken daily, Zyprexa. Sometimes, if I cannot sleep, I take Klonopin, but that kind of time is rare. Since being diagnosed with severe mental illness, I have tried at least seven medicines. I have taken at least one medicine specifically for depression, and it helped very much, but I don't remember its name. I don't take it now. The general consensus of my family is that nothing else has worked for me as well as Zyprexa. Nearly all the antipsychotics but Geodon did something to help me.

Barnaby, 23: Currently, I am taking three psychotropic medications. I have been prescribed a fair cross-section of antipsychotics, from Risperdal to Zyprexa to Serzone. There was nothing wrong with any of them; they just didn't do as much good as Clozaril.

Harriet, 43: I take Zyprexa, Mellaril, generic Paxil, Klonopin, Neurontin, and birth control. I have probably been on at least 20 medications. Zyprexa and Mellaril are very good. Lamictal gave me strong, vivid flashbacks that made me very unstable.

Ozzie, 46: I'm only on perphenazine. I was on olanzapine in the hospital. Both drugs worked well.

Larry, 46: One now, and 15 - 20 overall. Clozaril and lithium.

Jill, 27: Clozaril, Lamictal, Cymbalta, Klonopin.

Aileen, 54: I am on two psychotropic meds now. I have tried five or six. These two have been acceptable. The others were not acceptable.

Antipsychotic medications have been available since the 1950s. All of the antipsychotics affect neurotransmitters in the brain and all block dopamine receptors. They also affect other neurotransmitters to varying degrees. Side effects of the different medicines vary considerably, and can be quite troubling for some people. There are now many available medicines and it is very difficult to predict who will respond to which medicine. Only one medicine, clozapine, has been consistently shown to work better when other medicines do not work well.

Black Madonna, 36: Two. Twenty or more. Depakote – some antidepressants made me experience mania.

Christen, 44: I do not know the names of the medications I am on now. My husband is in charge of fixing it for me and going to the pharmacy. He does a good job.

Brian, 43: I am only on one at present. Since I got sick, I have been on at least six other medications and none of them worked as well for me as Clozaril has.

Jay, 56: I'm taking about four or five psychotropic medications. I've probably tried about a dozen. All were acceptable at the time, although none stopped the psychotic episodes from occurring.

Liana, 50: Four—I've tried about five medications since I developed mental illness. Cogentin and empirin codeine #3 were acceptable.

Have you ever not taken your medication? What happened? Is this currently an issue?

Jade, 43: I always think about not taking my meds. I always take my meds. It will always be an issue for me.

Socrates, 43: I stopped taking my meds several times, either because the side-effects were unbearable or I thought I was healed. Every time I became manic and psychotic and ended up hospitalized. Non-compliance is no longer an issue.

Adam, 28: I don't think about not taking my meds. When I don't take them, I get light-headed.

Danny Green, 46: Never.

Brunhilda, 44: I almost always take my medication. I've learned my lesson about not taking it. When I forget it, the results vary from medication to medication. On my current medication, it only sets me back about two weeks, and the symptoms don't become permanent.

Zelda, 48: No. Part of the reason why I take my meds is that, it is either take them or go back to Dorothea Dix hospital and get a shot of Haldol. This is not currently an issue.

> Many people have difficulty facing the prospect of taking medication for the rest of their lives, and therefore going off medication is the single greatest reason for relapse and hospitalization. Approximately 70% of patients (50% outpatient/ 20% inpatient) cease taking medication by the second year following their first hospitalization (Torrey 293).

Will, 38: I only forget doses on occasion. Sometimes I am slack about going to the pharmacy. Once I forgot my meds on a long weekend trip, but this did not create a significant problem.

Jane, 53: Once because of horrible sensitivity to heat, I went for a long time without taking Seroquel, the medicine I was on then. I eventually had what people call a relapse, and my family put me in the hospital. It still took a lot of lecturing and coaxing for the hospital people to get me to take medicine voluntarily. During that hospital stay, my doctor decided to change my medicine, so the immediate problem was solved. I have not since gone for a long time without taking my daily dose of medicine. Nevertheless, taking Zyprexa, I am frightened of getting diabetes, so frightened that I am sometimes tempted to stop taking the medicine. If I start getting sick, I think I can guarantee that that is going to be an issue. I am not so frightened of getting sick if I stop the Zyprexa, especially since being assured that the Lord can forgive me what is past. Nevertheless, when I tried the Geodon, I practically had a nervous breakdown, so I feel properly cautious at this point.

Barnaby, 23: At one point I was taking liquid Risperdal. One night I poured out the medicine and refilled the bottles with water. My symptoms came back with renewed force. I'll never do that again.

Harriet, 43: Yes, frank psychosis. It is not currently an issue.

Larry, 46: Yes, my symptoms began to get worse to where they would become unbearable. No.

Aileen, 54: Yes, one summer I didn't take my meds. I began to hear voices again and some magical thinking. I had to go back to the hospital. This is not currently an issue.

Black Madonna, 36: Unfortunately, I stopped taking my meds on two occasions, and paid big time for that – I had an episode. I now faithfully take my medication. This is not currently an issue.

Christen, 44: One time I thought I was better and didn't take it and had a relapse.

Brian, 43: Yes, when I do not take it I get sick again rather quickly. This is no longer an issue.

Jay, 56: Yes, in the past I've stopped my meds, which caused a severe decompensation. I have not stopped taking my meds in about 15 or 20 years.

Rachel, 44: Every time I take less than 10mg of Haldol, my thinking becomes distorted. Not taking my medicine is not an issue because the medicine is, above all, greatly helpful.

Liana, 50: After February of 1979 my mother said, "Shouldn't you be taking your medicine?"

What are the common side effects of these drugs, which you absolutely refuse to tolerate? What is the worst side effect you do tolerate?

Jade, 43: I would not accept diabetes. The worst side effect is the weight gain.

Socrates, 43: I will not tolerate tardive dyskinesia, tremors, akathisia. In the past I have tolerated dry mouth. I have no real side-effects with my present meds, except occasional diarrhea.

Adam, 28: None. Restlessness.

Danny Green, 46: I refuse to tolerate any of the doz-

> **Tardive dyskinesia** refers to the involuntary movements that often look like tics and come from prolonged use of some antipsychotic medications. Common movements include blinking and lip-smacking (en.wikipedia.org/wiki/Tardive_dyskinesia).

ens of failures. Currently, because they are working, I can tolerate anything.

Brunhilda, 44: I refuse to take antipsychotics that cause akathisia, such as Haldol. It is an awful side effect, worse than a panic attack. What I do tolerate is extreme weight gain, eczema, inability to swallow, and at the same time, dry mouth (imagine that!) and a weak bladder.

Zelda, 48: Weight gain and fatigue. This fatigue thing may be due to age.

Will, 38: Weight gain—Zyprexa. Tardive dyskinesia, stiffness, and rigidity, unsteady hands—Haldol and others. There were times when I was very conscious of my unsteady fingers and hands, barely able to write a check.

Jane, 53: The worst side effect I do tolerate is the difficulty losing weight with Zyprexa.

Barnaby, 23: Thankfully, Clozaril doesn't cause tardive dyskinesia. I don't have to worry about that (that's horrible stuff, too). When I took my medications twice a day, I slept all day and gained some weight. All in all, though, taking the medication is worth it.

Harriet, 43: Lamictal gave me flashbacks that I could not tolerate. I do tolerate weight gain and dry mouth.

Ozzie, 46: No side effects.

Jill, 27: Weight gain—I tolerate it but I do try and watch my diet and exercise. Sometimes headaches.

Aileen, 54: I refuse to tolerate feeling dead. Constipa-

> **Akathisia,** a common side effect of antipsychotic medications, can make a person feel like they have to keep moving. It can range from a mild discomfort to feelings of anxiety and restlessness (en.wikipedia.org/wiki/Akathisia).

tion and lack of sexual desire are the worst of the side effects I now have.

Black Madonna, 36: I absolutely refuse to tolerate weight gain – tremors.

Brian, 43: The worst side effect of my current medication is a strong sedative effect which causes me to sleep a lot. But I do tolerate it.

Jay, 56: There are none. The worst side-effect is sexual impotency.

Rachel, 44: I cannot tolerate extreme insomnia or extreme sleepiness.

Liana, 50: I won't tolerate violent illness. I took iron pills, and they were constipating. I feel like iron is tolerable.

Elaborations...

Socrates, 43: The first medicine I was ever put on was Haldol, which caused me more suffering than my illness at the time. It caused me to break out in hives and lose some of my hair, but the worst side effect was what I can only describe as a feeling that I was crawling out of my skin. I had constant unrest and anguish and a feeling similar to what they now call "restless leg syndrome," except that my whole body was affected. I suffered on this med for six months until my doctor took me off it. I later discovered that I was allergic to Haldol.

Barnaby, 23: In my case, the negative symptoms had more destructive power on my life than the positive ones, so I tried to imbue myself with the social skills I had lost. Unfortunately, I found that endeavor impossible; it was my medication that changed things. There was nothing I could have done on my own. After my medicine started helping, that's when I found I had to practice my social skills, and I still am practicing. I think it's extremely important to be around people, preferably people you can trust, to relearn how to be well.

Hospitals, Therapies and Clubhouses

We have met the enemy, and he is us.

— Walt Kelly

Poem for Progress

– Claudia Moon

I
Imagine robots on skateboards
bumping into each other's shadows.

II
It's we I speak of
on our appointed hallway
for at least 72 hours.

III
Bumping into each other,
bumping into each other's shadows.
Different diagnoses.
The same pathos.
A loss of self.
The blending of boundaries.
Lips chalky with medication.
Arms stiff from side effects.

IV
There is no value in saying
"excuse me," we know
there is no purpose
in any collision.

V
Bones and bodies
carry the exhaustion
of horrifying images, the
constant strain of words
attacking, the floors
shifting below with
no pattern.

VI
Our knocking bones
recognize these traits
within one another, familiar
like blood cousins, going
in no real direction.

VII
We push past each other,
Heading for the same place.

Can you describe your experience with hospitalization?

Jade, 43: 1997-2000 in and out, revolving door. 2000-2003, state hospital.

Socrates, 43: I have been hospitalized 13 times, but not at all in the last seven years; some of these have involved great suffering, all have involved some suffering. I remember my first hospitalization vividly. At first I thought the staff were devil worshipers and were going to sacrifice me to the devil, so I tried to escape. I broke a thick door window laced with metal (which was supposed to be unbreakable) but found that the door had no doorknobs. Orderlies raced toward me and I picked up some shattered glass and waved them off. A nurse told me to drop the glass, and I remember resigning to the fact that I would be sacrificed and dropped the glass. I was placed in a padded room, and a doctor came in and sutured my wounds. His good humor made me realize that these people were here to help me, and this realization began my recovery.

Adam, 28: Difficult. Humbling to witness other people's struggles.

Danny Green, 46: From ages 16-21 years I was mostly in hospitals. Some were better than the streets or "home." Some were worse.

> Hospitalization is currently reserved for emergencies, in which it is determined that patients are a danger to themselves or others. The majority of hospitalizations are now only a few days to a few weeks (Smith 8,9).

Brunhilda, 44: One time when I was not suicidal, I went into the hospital for three weeks for a medication change. I gained 50 pounds without knowing it or anyone noticing. I later gained even more. I must be the only one to admit I liked the food at the time.

Zelda, 48: Constantly being told what to do. Regulation of life. Smoking of cigarettes.

Will, 38: Manic flight to NYC—stay at St. Luke's in Manhattan. In-patient stays or "going on vacation" as I come to call it, were usually helpful over time.

Jane, 53: That could take a book. People used to be much more polite than they have seemed lately sometimes, but fortunately, that is not universally true. Hospital people have generally been very gentle and considerate, or at least concerned, when I was suicidal, and that helped a lot. Once, for a protracted time, I had a roommate who was very frightened of the nurses and various attendants during her hospital stay, and that was hard for me. Once or twice, the nurses brought enforcers with them to give me medicine that they were determined I was going to take, and that made quite an impression, which was not altogether positive. I was not threatening anybody when that happened. Once, I was put in another institution than UNC Hospital for a while, but I think that was my fault. When I was transferred to UNC, I soon felt better.

Barnaby, 23: I've been to three different inpatient programs on six or seven separate occasions. The first time was after a suicide attempt. I tell you, which facility you go to makes a big difference—the difference between being relatively stress-free for a few days and being a prisoner watching the world pass by.

Ozzie, 46: It gave me time to rethink what I was going through. I was working so hard in construction, and it was nice to be babied.

Larry, 46: I was hospitalized about 20 times both state and private. They started being unbearable until I started to allow them to help.

Jill, 27: Most of my hospitalizations were when I was 16 and 17. They were positive in that I got on the right medication and a correct diagnosis. My recent hospitalization in March, 2006, was not so pleasant.

Aileen, 54: I was on UNC 3rd floor two different times. I mostly enjoyed my time there. People were friendly—both patients and staff.

> Hospitalization can be helpful in diagnosing and determining treatments. The patient's behavior and reactions to medications are observed by the staff. The hospital also provides a structured and safe environment (Smith 9).

Black Madonna, 36: Yes! I have been hospitalized about 10 times. I always like to go to the hospital—there is never a resistance. The doctors and nurses at UNC are really knowledgeable. They are good people.

Christen, 44: I have been hospitalized at least 10 times already.

Brian, 43: I was hospitalized for the first time in 1986 and was in and out of the state hospital for about two years. Then I got into a university hospital and was in and out of it for about four years.

Jay, 56: For the most part I've found hospitalizations to have been beneficial. With the exception of one early in my history, all have been helpful.

Liana, 50: I was violently ill.

What do you like about the hospital? What do you dislike?

Jade, 43: When I am really sick, it keeps me safe. I hate to be locked up.

Socrates, 43: I have had some positive experiences in hospitals. Sometimes there is a feeling of comfort, but I do not like losing my freedom. I also wish most hospitals would provide more outside and recreational time.

Adam, 28: Stabilizing effect. Too long a stay.

Danny Green, 46: The chance to adjust to medicine in a safe environment. The chance of abuse by staff towards inpatients can be realized behind locked doors.

Brunhilda, 44: Another time, when I was depressed, I went in the hospital thinking I would sit around and feel sorry for myself. Big surprise! There were so many activities, therapies, and appointments, I never had the chance to focus on my depression or problems. That's a very good thing about the hospital!

Zelda, 48: Nothing. Everything.

Will, 38: As an inpatient, I could get away from my parents. However, inpatient stays would make me rather paranoid at times, especially when I was not doing well.

Jane, 53: That could take a book! I like kindness when I encounter it, and I have had several very profitable and curing hospitalizations, related to physical problems. When I encounter rudeness or mockery, I dislike it very much. I also like it that there are nourishing meals there, and that there are many doctors who care very much about their patients. Of course, I dislike that a hospital stay can be expensive, but Medicaid has helped with that tremendously.

Barnaby, 23: A hospital can be an escape. Sometimes I felt a little better just being there. But a hospital can be torture, too. I used to get cabin fever, and that actually made my symptoms worse. There was so little to do, all I could do was get lost in my head.

Ozzie, 46: I liked the activities like art and sports and developing new friendships. I disliked being treated like a prisoner.

Larry, 46: The opportunity to get out, having to start over when you get out.

Jill, 27: I like that they can adjust my medications quickly—I dislike being locked up because I have abandonment issues.

Aileen, 54: I liked the regular schedule. I disliked having to ask for my meds.

Black Madonna, 36: I liked recreation time, arts and crafts, and watching TV.

Christen, 44: I didn't like some of the activities they made me do, especially the games. I liked talking with the nurses – they made me feel better.

UNC's inpatient unit has a variety of services available: **psychiatric treatment** that focuses on the stabilization of symptoms; **social work**, providing individualized case management, discharge planning, and family counseling; **occupational therapy** providing evaluations of functional ability and programs like cooking groups, coping skills, independent living skills, and one-on-one discharge planning; and **recreational therapy** providing individualized assessments and treatment plans to improve overall functioning in leisure, cognitive, and physical domains (www.psychiatry.unc.edu/STEP/step.htm). A typical hospital stay is three-to-five days.

Brian, 43: I liked the feeling of safety and comfort. I did not like being locked up and restrained from normal freedoms such as going outside for a walk or a drive in the car.

Jay, 56: A safe place where I can get a reduction in symptoms. I disliked being confined, but it was necessary.

Rachel, 44: I like the camaraderie in the hospital with other patients. I feel safe and protected in the hospital. I dislike the lack of exercise, and the fact that I nearly always gain weight in the hospital.

Liana, 50: Ping pong and other games are enjoyable. Having to take pills that cause suffering is my major complaint. Also, I disliked it when they said I weighed 30 lbs. less than my actual weight.

If you're a clubhouse member, what do you like about the clubhouse? What do you dislike?

Jade, 43: I like working at the thrift shop. I don't like a lot of hanging around.

> Clubhouses focus on helping people with severe mental illness with employment, housing and socialization. The Fountain House in New York developed a model program in the 1950s and has now accredited over 400 clubhouses worldwide (Anderson 13). One hallmark of the clubhouse model is voluntary participation.

Socrates, 43: I enjoy social interaction at the clubhouse while smoking on the porch. Sometimes, however, some people are verbally combative, but only one or two people ever act antisocial.

Danny Green, 46: One-on-one relationships. Too many people.

Zelda, 48: I am a clubhouse member and my relation to the clubhouse is complex. Dislike? The professionalism.

Will, 38: When a clubhouse member, I never really visited much, except to get a decent, hot, cheap meal. The clubhouse I belonged to tended to over-stimulate me and was quite crowded.

Jane, 53: I have never really liked the clubhouse very much or felt that I needed it dreadfully, but I like it for those who like it and who use it much more than I do. It must be very hard to be a clubhouse worker and face the budget cuts, laws, and institutional rules with which such a worker has to cope.

Harriet, 43: I am a clubhouse member for a year. I love my friends, seeing others' illnesses and feeling like I belong. I dislike the pressure to "engage" more in the clubhouse work—it makes me very anxious.

Larry, 46: They gave me an opportunity to be employed. Nothing.

Jill, 27: I love the socialization. I like the structure. I don't like that they call it adult day care, and sometimes I wish there was time for more in-clubhouse social activities.

Aileen, 54: I like the thrift shop and seeing my friends there. I dislike the chaos I find there and trying to fit in.

Black Madonna, 36: I like social events – just getting together with the other members, and having lots of fun. I like working in the Admin Unit and sometimes, cooking and serving. There is nothing I dislike at this time.

Christen, 44: I like answering the phones and doing things under the administrative unit. I love everyone in the clubhouse. All my best friends go to the clubhouse.

Brian, 43: I am a very active clubhouse member. What I like about the clubhouse is the opportunities it offers, and the socialization and relationships.

Jay, 56: I am a clubhouse member and what I like is the social experience. The thing I dislike is not enough interaction with staff.

Rachel, 44: In the past I did not feel that my abilities and time were well used in the clubhouse. I have heard very good things about one of the clubhouses in this area, but live too far away to make use of it.

Liana, 50: The other club house members are bright and compassionate. The staff is ingenious and empathetic. I thoroughly enjoy all socials. Most of the time I just like to be lazy in my apartment, but I do janitorial work an hour a day, which I dislike.

Have you had problems getting along with others who have mental illness in the hospital? the clubhouse? or in the community?

Socrates, 43: Once a roommate went ballistic and threw a bed at me while in the hospital. In the clubhouse a certain individual is accusatory and verbally combative at times, but he's like that with everyone, and I realize he has issues. I have no problems in the community at large.

Brunhilda, 44: The main problem I have getting along with other people with mental illness is their reading things into what is not there, and taking everything personally, even if it wasn't meant that way.

Will, 38: These days I relate to most anyone rather well. Good interpersonal social skills have come with time, effort, education, and active listening efforts.

Jane, 53: I have not really had a significant problem getting along with someone in the hospital. In the clubhouse, one member said he liked me and then talked about committing suicide, which frightened me terribly, so I stayed away and spent a lot of time praying for him since he seemed much more dependent on the clubhouse than I was. I don't think I have problems dealing with anyone in the community. I did have a bit of an argument with a pharmacist once, before I understood what he was trying to tell me; since then there has been no trouble at the pharmacy, and I am grateful for their help.

Barnaby, 23: There were a few patients that creeped me out but were nice to me. Only one patient really got me mad—so I avoided her. More often than not, I get along with people who have mental illness. It's almost a subculture that's nice to be accepted into. My best buddy and I met in a hospital.

Ozzie, 46: In the hospital, one patient called me a blue-eyed mother-f, and he would jab me with pens, and one time punched me in the jaw.

Black Madonna, 36: No, I am an easy person to get along with—I have tried to treat everyone I know with a mental illness with respect and dignity.

Christen, 44: Sometimes I have disagreements with others, but we always make up.

Brian, 43: Sometimes it is hard to get along with people when they are sick or not doing well.

Rachel, 44: I find I have extra compassion for others with mental illness and that they have compassion for me.

Liana, 50: Yes—the guy that lives in the apartments keeps asking, "Why won't you be my girlfriend?" and he keeps touching me.

Which types of therapies have you participated in?

Jade, 43: Cognitive behavioral therapy; group therapy; individual social work consultations. They helped me with my perceptions, get a fresh look on things.

Socrates, 43: I have only engaged in individual psychotherapy with a doctor.

Adam, 28: Individual psychotherapy.

Brunhilda, 44: Cognitive behavioral therapy for two years helped me by changing my thought systems. It really changed my life. Group therapy—all of us are female, most have the same diagnosis and are a similar age. I can compare with these women and don't feel so alone. Social work consultation—I reserve these for helping me with the system red tape and socialization. There is so much of this I need help with.

Zelda, 48: Occupational therapy, cognitive behavioral therapy and dialectical behavioral therapy with my regular therapist. Group therapy, workshops, and social work consultations.

Will, 38: Occupational therapy and recreational therapy, inpatient, something to do. Psychotherapy, invaluable. I would have been lost without it.

Jane, 53: I have participated a little in occupational therapy, which has encouraged me for seeking a job. Concerning group therapy, I was once in a physical education group, from which I learned some handy barbell exercises.

Barnaby, 23: When it comes to individual therapy, finding an understanding therapist is important. I've had therapists that actually made me feel bad over my symptoms. These days I leave therapy feeling pretty good about myself. I think group therapy is great because you get to relate to the people with you when you can't relate to anyone else.

Harriet, 43: For three years in dialectical behavioral therapy group, and for 30 years in individual therapy.

Ozzie, 46: Group therapy, workshops, and individual psychotherapy.

Larry, 46: Group therapy and individual psychotherapy.

Jill, 27: Occupational therapy—at the hospital—not helpful. Dialectical behavioral therapy group—yes, it was helpful. Social work consultation—helpful. Individual psychotherapy—helpful.

Aileen, 54: Occupational thearpy—in hospital, group activities. Cognitive behavioral therapy—helped me structure my time. Dialectical behavioral therapy—helped me learn to cope and make friends. Group therapy—let me be in touch with women with similar obstacles. Individual social work consultation—helped with everyday and long-term projects. Individual psychotherapy—helped with everyday and long-term problems.

Black Madonna, 36: Group therapy at the Mental Health Association for people who have bipolar, and the STEP Clinic. Individual psychotherapy—I am in a personal program called Attacking Anxiety and Depression, which is cognitive behavioral therapy.

Christen, 44: I liked occupational therapy because I like to make things. I also liked group therapy but I no longer participate. Most of all, I love my social worker and see her every week.

Brian, 43: The things that have helped me the most are medication and the clubhouse. I have used occupational thearpy, workshops, social work consultations, and individual therapy.

Jay, 56: Occupational therapy, cognitive behavioral therapy, group therapy, individual social work consultations, individual therapy.

Rachel, 44: Cognitive behavioral therapy, group therapy, and individual therapy.

Liana, 50: Group therapy—participated in enjoyable social games in 1987. My social worker weighs me once a week to show me that someone cares. In group therapy in 1987, I felt recognized.

Elaborations...

Danny, Green 46: As a teenager, I spent a year as a psychiatric inpatient at the Medical College of Virginia. This is a public facility in Richmond. Much of the time I stayed within the confines of the Intensive Care Unit. It sounds oppressive, but it proved a decidedly good and caring environment. Ms. C. worked as a nurse there. She was an angel. Mr. S., Ms. C., Mr. H., and all the staff were terrific.

I played mock football in the hallways with my friends and fellow patients, Teddy "Red" and Dwayne. My sister Julia brought me three LPs, which I played constantly inside the ward on my white plastic GE record player. They were "After the Gold Rush," by Neil Young, an anthology, "Flowers," by the Rolling Stones, and "The Freewheelin' Bob Dylan."

I met beautiful people named Margaret and Wayne. I played ping-pong with Chester. I had two fine public school tutors who visited me on the ward. Larry B. taught me English. Rosalee B. taught me the history of the Russian revolution.

The doctors at M.C.V. were essentially quacks, but they honored the Hippocratic Oath and did no harm. They never prescribed me harsh neuroleptics.

In contrast stands the Northern Virginia Mental Health Hospital on Gallows Road in Fairfax, VA. I was force-fed tranquilizers there which made me very sick indeed. Because these drugs damaged my mind so badly, the staff periodically locked me in "quiet rooms," while I tried steadily to recover my sanity from its battle with the drugs' toxicity. Three times I underwent electric shock therapy at a neighboring facility. My despair grew so deep that I tried to take my life by jumping in front of a car on Gallows Road.

At no time did my doctors ask me how their drugs made me feel. My own testimony had no value to them. They ignored it entirely. The obscenely observational approach towards our diagnosis so typical of the 20th-Century psychiatry won out over any of our objections.

There were also all types of legal proceedings happening around us. Unqualified doctors consorting with equally unqualified lawyers were all painting the picture of an unqualified farce. The welfare of the patients lagged well behind any priority set by these hearings. We were written off as too incompetent to testify.

Jade, 43: I've been brought in chained and shackled. I have walked in voluntarily. I tried to run. I've asked for more time. The defining factor underlying my hospitalizations is that hospitals are here to save lives. Even in the harsh environment of the state hospital, safety is the bottom line.

Connecting with hospital staff members can be life changing. In smaller community hospitals or plush private hospitals you stand a better chance of connecting with staff and talking through some of your struggles. I have been given back my will to live in hospitals; and yet, never have I felt so utterly alone as in a hospital.

I have felt judged in hospitals. In hospitals I have felt redeemed. The best thing a hospital can do when you are ill is not to be threatening, supervise self-destructive tendencies, give you time to get better, and always convey a trust in your inner core.

In the state hospital it was wise to align yourself with hateful people so those same people wouldn't single you out as a target. Peer groups in hospitals range from downright scary (criminals and sociopaths) to very supportive friendships.

The physical constructions I've experienced range from prison-like conditions to private hospitals with plush rooms and good food. When you are really sick you don't notice your environment that much, although I'm sure it influences your emotional state.

In order to survive being hospitalized you learn to mind your own business and work on getting better each day. Don't depend on staff or doctors to make you better. It must come from you.

Mental Health Professionals

Whenever a doctor cannot do good, he must keep from doing harm.

– Hippocrates

I Cry

– Barnaby

I cry to speak
I cry to swear
I cry for lovers never there
I cry for you
I cry to do
I cry to wash my face
I cry the smiles and the laughter
I cry the empty space

I cry for me
I cry to see
I cry to picture all my fears
If crying started with a laugh
And ended more than tears
I'd cry to sing like happy kings
I'd cry to try with angel wings

What type of outpatient professionals do you see, and how frequently do you see them?

Jade, 43: I see a doctor about once a month, a group once a week, and a social worker once a week.

Socrates, 43: I see my psychiatrist every three months.

Adam, 28: Psychotherapist twice a month; doctor once every two months.

Danny Green, 46: Social work, once weekly.

Brunhilda, 44: I see my resident and attending psychiatrists once a month, my social worker once a month, and I try to go to group therapy three times a month.

Zelda, 48: I see my therapist once a week and my doctor once a month.

Will, 38: Med checks with the doctor every three months (or longer).

Jane, 53: I see two psychiatrists, one a resident and one a professor and specialist in medicines, sometimes once a month, and sometimes more or less frequently, depending on whether I am changing medicines or suffering from side effects related to them.

Barnaby, 23: I see my therapist every week and my psychiatrist once a month.

Harriet, 43: Psychiatrist once a week.

Ozzie, 46: I see a resident physician at UNC Hospital. I see him every six weeks.

Larry, 46: Psychiatrist—every 6 months.

Jill, 27: My psychiatrist—every two weeks. My therapist—once a week. DBT group every week.

Aileen, 54: Social worker, twice a month. Counselor, once a month. Psychiatrist, once a month. Group, four times a month.

Black Madonna, 36: STEP Clinic every three months.

Christen, 44: I see my psychiatrist every two months and my social worker once a week.

Brian, 43: I see my psychiatrist once every four months and have daily interactions with clubhouse staff.

Jay, 56: I see an MSW for individual therapy; I see an MSW for group therapy; I see a resident in psychiatry for medication.

Liana, 50: I see my social worker once a week and a psychiatrist once a month.

What do you like and dislike about your treatment team?

Jade, 43: It's just enough to keep me going. Sometimes I miss my therapist in Kansas.

Socrates, 43: My doctor is receptive and supportive.

Adam, 28: Like it, effective.

Danny Green, 46: I like everything about my doctors and social worker.

Brunhilda, 44: I like that everyone on my treatment team has a specific function and communicates with each other. What I dislike is when I tell something important to a treatment team member, and I want the whole team to know, and they don't pass it on. Even though everyone has their specialties, you may end up telling everyone the same thing. I always ask the same questions to everyone because I receive different information from the different positions (such as side effects).

Zelda, 48: I like them. Dislike: none.

Will, 38: I do believe that a comprehensive treatment team is a most effective, best evidence-based practice to keep mental health consumers in the community.

Jane, 53: I like my resident psychiatrist very much. I can talk with her about practically anything when I see her, and I have been very open and frank with her. The professor, of course, I appreciate for his expertise and, I have learned, for his openness in dealing with new information. Sometimes I think that dealing with patients has inured him to reports of all the side effects that we suffer. I wish that there were something more to deal with these side effects. Sometimes with a hard side effect or two and in the desperate mental state which I reached, I got very angry and concluded that the specialist in drugs did not care about what I suffered, but I am willing to consider that my opinion might have been wrong. I generally get along with specialists, although my experiences with medicines have sometimes been difficult.

Barnaby, 23: I like that they really know what they're doing. With therapy I can get stuff off my chest that I can't disclose to anyone else for fear they won't want to be around me any more.

Harriet, 43: When I get depressed, I feel alone.

Ozzie, 46: Sometimes they don't like my wife to come in to treatment. I like that they are looking out for my best interests.

Jill, 27: My psychiatrist is fair and doesn't like hospitals and does everything he can to help me. My therapist listens to me. DBT teaches me skills I need to have healthy friendships and deal with stress.

Aileen, 54: Social worker tries hard and really cares. Counselor sometimes seems to disapprove of my choices. Psychiatrist—ok—I like the attending more and wish I could see her more. Group is good.

Black Madonna, 36: I like the STEP Clinic, and sometimes talking with the social worker. I only wish I could keep the same doctor for a long period of time.

Christen, 44: I like everyone on my treatment team. I appreciate them working together so well to help me.

Jay, 56: No dislikes—I think it is very good.

Liana, 50: I like that they are friendly and encouraging.

Have you had misunderstandings or conflicts with your mental healthcare professionals? Explain.

Jade, 43: I am able to bring them up and deal with them as they come up.

Socrates, 43: Once in a hospital, a doctor refused to put me on my preferred med, so I refused to talk to him until he told me he wanted to talk to me about my discharge. I perked up then.

Brunhilda, 44: I haven't had a misunderstanding or conflict with anyone on my treatment team in a very long time. When I do, it is usually my social worker who intervenes for me. At least she will define the problem and double check whether or not I'm being rational about the conflict.

Zelda, 48: None. My therapist and I understand one another.

Will, 38: Rarely. As an inpatient, when very ill, I was particularly adept at escaping from a locked ward and walking home from the hospital.

Jane, 53: When I am taking a medicine and suffering from a side effect without relief, I can get very testy and sometimes angry. I have also explained why I feel like a prisoner of the medical establishment. That feeling continues.

Larry, 46: I had a doctor tell me he could relate to my illness, and I told him he may be able to understand it, but he sure as hell couldn't relate to it.

Aileen, 54: I used a certain med for a female problem, and my counselor let me know she disapproved by the sound of her voice. We didn't discuss her feelings.

Christen, 44: One psychiatrist wouldn't give me the medicine I thought I needed, but he did after I cussed him out.

Brian, 43: I had one conflict with a social worker at a state hospital who did not want to help me get out of the hospital, and I eventually had to arrange my own discharge and plan where I would go after leaving the hospital.

Jay, 56: Yes I have. One telling me that there was no legal protection in the mental health system. I walked out and reported her to the licensing authority, who investigated.

Liana, 50: I keep asking my psychiatrist that I see monthly if I can have amphetamines, and he repeatedly refuses to let me take them.

Which classification of mental healthcare professions or clubhouse staff are the most empathetic to your situation. Why do you think so?

Jade, 43: The doctor, the social worker, and the clubhouse caseworker are all very sensitive to my needs.

Socrates, 43: Of healthcare professionals, I have only had interactions with psychiatrists, but I am thinking of having therapy sessions with a social worker. Most of the clubhouse staff have been supportive and affirming.

Adam, 28: Psychotherapist—he's compassionate.

Danny Green, 46: Social worker—she's educated.

Brunhilda, 44: I love social workers. They seem genuinely interested in helping us with negative symptoms, socialization, job coaching, and helping us with the system. They treat us as a whole person, helping us solve our special challenges in life.

Zelda, 48: My therapist because I can demonstrate the dimensions of the problem.

Will, 38: Skilled psychotherapists. Mental health consumers need people who can really listen and provide useful feedback.

Jane, 53: I think that they all have the limitation that they are just not in the same body as I am and don't feel what I feel. Nevertheless, they all try to understand, and I hope I generally give them credit for that. I am beginning to get along very well with my psychiatry resident, and I am thankful for that. She may be the most empathetic of the professionals who deal with me. I am saying that because I can confide in her things I cannot yet confide in any other mental healthcare professional.

Barnaby, 23: I think therapists are most empathetic because they get to know you better and they have experience. They understand better because they've seen it before.

Harriet, 43: MSWs are the most empathetic.

Ozzie, 46: The attending doctor at UNC. He seems to understand me well.

Larry, 46: Clubhouse staff since they see members daily and have a chance to know them over time.

Jill, 27: My therapist because he sees me every week, and he really listens and gives me feedback.

Aileen, 54: The social worker, the counselor, and the attending physician are the most empathetic. They seem to understand most.

Black Madonna, 36: The STEP Clinic social worker. Each staff member is very caring and concerned about my welfare. They have even visited me at my home in time of crisis.

Christen, 44: My social worker and a person on the clubhouse staff are some of my favorite people because they help me so much.

Brian, 43: I think the clubhouse staff are because I see them five days a week and I know them and have an equal relationship with them and we have known each other for years.

Jay, 56: The therapist—it's part of their personality.

Rachel, 44: It really depends on the individual, how open-minded and intelligent they are, and how empathetic and non-judgmental.

Liana, 50: The classification of mental health care professionals that are the most empathetic are my social worker I see weekly, and three members of the Club Nova staff. They are cheerful and insightful, and they are my best friends.

Elaborations...

Will, 38: MDs are obsessed with treating symptoms and stabilizing meds. They seem to forget that mania can be a hell of a lot of fun. Pretty much everyone experiences depression at some point, and everyone likes to dream, but for those with labels, they are called delusions. Thank God that true love, passion and romance are not in the DSM-IV. It seems that everything else is, or has been at some time.

Support Systems: Relationships And Spirituality

Friend: One who knows all about you and loves you just the same.

– Elbert Hubbard

The Shepherd's Fold

— Mike Dunne

The closer I draw into the Light
The more refined my second sight
If others could see what I see
They would believe the same as me

That God sees all from His mighty throne
That man is truly not alone
That mercy awaits at the open door
That our souls survive, our spirits soar

Into the heavens or into the deep
This is a truth that I will keep
Safe from the thieves who would seek
To rob me of my priceless peace

But I cannot prove what my eyes have seen
Some think it is a madman's dream
But I know better, and to this I hold
I cannot be torn from the Shepherd's fold

The Serpent tried to steal my soul
Laid a snare to take control
But God for me had another plan
For I was spared by the Son of Man

He bore my sin, He bore my pain
He healed my soul, He healed my brain
He stayed with me through thick and thin
He triumphed over death and sin

And so to Him I owe my life
Purchased by His great sacrifice
And always His face I will behold
I cannot be torn from the Shepherd's Fold.

How did your parents originally react to your diagnosis/ illness? How do they react now?

Jade, 43: They were very scared. They learned all they could. They are more confident in my health now.

Socrates, 43: My parents were originally devastated by my illness. They did not understand it and were both greatly concerned for my well-being and yet fearful of me. My mother is deceased, but my father has become very supportive of me, though he still does not understand mental illness very well.

Adam, 28: Mom's guilt. Ignorance now.

Danny Green, 46: Blame and guilt. Differently and indifferently.

Brunhilda, 44: My mother was extremely guilt-tripped because my illness is genetic. I don't understand why—no one chooses their genes. To me, genetics is a no-blame situation. I put my mother through so much that now she is finally happy with me because I am so much better now and the worst is over.

Zelda, 48: We had just arrived here after a repatriation. To keep it short, they were sad. I don't know what they thought of Dorothea Dix Hospital.

Will, 38: Then: father denied; mother proactive. Now: father, sensitive, discreet; mother, proud and supportive.

Jane, 53: My parents generally believe everything the psychiatrists tell them. They were not surprised when originally told I had schizoaffective disorder, and they were not surprised when told that it was probably lifelong.

Barnaby, 23: My dad never accepted that I was sick. Even when my symptoms were at their worst, he denied I had any illness. My mom wanted to believe I wasn't as sick as I was, saying that the voices I hear were due to my imagination. When I started to get better, my mom would say, "He's not sick any more." My dad would reply that I never was. I never did confide in them very much.

Harriet, 43: Initially they did not know what life I'd have. They are proud of me and support my treatment emotionally and financially.

Ozzie, 46: They are both gone.

Larry, 46: They have always been very supportive.

Jill, 27: Originally supportive but didn't know much. Now they are extremely active in the mental health awareness community, like NAMI.

Aileen, 54: My mother became very sympathetic to me and my life. She tried to help with the side effects. My father was deceased. My mother is now deceased.

Black Madonna, 36: They were supportive. Still supportive.

Christen, 44: My parents didn't understand and gave me a hard time at first. My mother cried. Now they're ok with it, that the worst part is over.

Brian, 43: They both reacted with anger and denial, and it has only changed in the sense that they are more tolerant and supportive of other aspects of my life.

Jay, 56: Concerned and caring. Both are deceased.

Rachel, 44: Originally it was to them as if the person that they had known had died. They still get frustrated that I can't "just snap out of it."

Liana, 50: My mother was heart-broken in 1976. My father said in 1987, "You have to eat," because a doctor kept saying I was anorexic.

How did your siblings originally react to your diagnosis/ illness? How do they react now?

Jade, 43: My brother doesn't want to talk about it.

Socrates, 43: My siblings, like my parents, originally reacted to my illness with fear. My sisters still do not understand it, but my brother does, and has become one of my greatest supporters.

Adam, 28: Blame. Now it's better.

Danny Green, 46: Concern, great compassion.

Brunhilda, 44: One of my sisters was in high school when I became ill. She didn't understand why I was getting so much attention from my parents, while she deserved the attention for being high-achieving. Now, she realizes that I needed more help in life than she did at the time.

Zelda, 48: Indifferent.

Will, 38: Then: brother, helpful, and sister, not around. Now: both are supportive and proud, sharing my commitment to wellness and life.

Jane, 53: I have at least one sibling who reacted very negatively when told that my illness was lifelong. I don't blame him. He doesn't want me to be a bother to him. I have reason to think that he does not want to be stuck doing reports on how I do with what resources I am given. I do not know in detail how the other siblings acted, but I know that at least one of them wants me to take my medicine without fail.

Barnaby, 23: My brother believes my illness is purely psychological. He and my sister never talk about my illness, but they don't look at me the same way they used to. It sucks.

Harriet, 43: I have an adopted brother, 37, who doesn't relate to me regarding my illness.

Ozzie, 46: They were sympathetic and helped me with my bills and credit cards. Now they don't mention my illness except on rare occasions.

Larry, 46: They have been very supportive.

Jill, 27: Originally my brother was like, "So what?" Now he is very supportive.

Aileen, 54: My sister worried about me and still does. She is as supportive as she knows how to be. My brother tries to "top" my problem with his.

Black Madonna, 36: Supportive. Still supportive.

Christen, 44: I have very little contact with my brothers and sister.

Brian, 43: I have two sisters. One of them reacted with sympathy, and the other reacted by being very supportive and actually joined NAMI and became very active in advocacy.

Jay, 56: Accepting, although not originally.

Rachel, 44: When I was having a major breakdown, my brother lamented, "I want my sister back." Now he is usually very supportive and seems to have a better understanding of my illness than most people do.

Liana, 50: My brother said, "I didn't like taking you to the hospital."

Does anyone else in your family have mental illness? What do you know about him or her?

Jade, 43: My cousin—bipolar. My aunt—electroconvulsive therapy (ECT).

Socrates, 43: My mother had schizophrenia, and my cousin (on her side of the family) also has schizophrenia. I know little about either because I never saw my mother after I was four years old (she has since died), and I have had no contact with my cousin since then. I only know about his illness from my uncle.

Danny Green, 46: Yes, my mother's sister died of it, falling prey to suicide at age 25.

Brunhilda, 44: My uncle has mental illness. It skipped a generation, and now my cousin's daughter has mental illness. My uncle is highly functioning and worked at a government position full-time for over 30 years.

Will, 38: Well, history of mental illness and substance abuse in my family not completely or effectively addressed.

Jane, 53: The only other "family member" who has mental illness is an aunt by marriage and therefore not related to me in the bloodline. When talked to ra-

Relative	Occurrence of Schizophrenia
No Ill Relative	1%
Ill Aunt or Uncle	3%
Ill Parent or Sibling	5 – 10%
Both Parents Ill	15 – 20%
Non-Identical Twin	5 – 10%
Identical Twin	25 – 45%
(Mueser and Gingrich 19)	

tionally and calmly, she can be quite reasonable and can even come through a crisis well.

Harriet, 43: Mother—depression.

Ozzie, 46: Yes, my younger brother. I don't know much about him.

Jill, 27: Deceased cousin. I only know he was bipolar and spent a good deal of time in hospitals. I have an uncle with bipolar. I have two more cousins with bipolar. My family doesn't talk much about them.

Aileen, 54: My cousin, age 19, has schizophrenia. It was years before she was diagnosed. She seems to be dealing well on the correct med.

Brian, 43: Yes, my mother has schizophrenia. She has had it since I was a child and still struggles to this day.

Rachel, 44: My mother had been diagnosed as schizoaffective and may also have been undiagnosed as bipolar. I regret that the understanding of mental illness was so poorly developed at that time in history.

Liana, 50: Yes, I had a great-aunt that had shock treatments.

How did or would your life change when your parents die(d)?

Jade, 43: I'll completely fall apart.

Socrates, 43: My mother's death when I was 19 years old was devastating because I had not seen her since I was four, and I was trying to find her at the time. Her death coincided with the onset of my illness, but was not the main factor in it. Now that I am more mature, I see death as just a transition to the next existence, and though I would be greatly saddened by my father's death, I take comfort in my faith that I will see him in the world to come.

Adam, 28: I was eight years old when I lost my dad. Major effect for a long time.

Danny Green, 46: I would miss them.

Brunhilda, 44: I rely on my mother all the time. I don't know what would happen between me and my siblings if she were to die. She is "the glue that binds" the family. My father died 10 years ago, and life has changed a lot. He was always angry at me. My father was a very logical person, and what he hated most was irrationality.

Zelda, 48: It would be devastating.

Will, 38: Sorrow and finances. I would miss both and feel sorry for both, for different reasons.

Jane, 53: If my parents died, I would miss them very much. I think that someone else in the family would assume authority over me, but I am not sure who would do this.

Barnaby, 23: I would have a ton of new-found responsibility. My mom helps me a lot with all sorts of day-to-day stuff. I'd have to learn quickly. Of course, I don't want to think of them dying, anyway.

Harriet, 43: It will be devastating. But I am protected by a will.

Ozzie, 46: I felt I had lost a great friend. I didn't have the support I once had.

Larry, 46: I would become even more dependent on clubhouse people and the opportunities they have provided me.

Jill, 27: I don't want to think about it.

Aileen, 54: I started flossing my teeth when my mother died, probably because she had dentures. I couldn't talk to her every day or get her help with problems. After eight years, I still grieve.

Black Madonna, 36: My life changed because my mother was special to me—there was a hole in my heart, I miss her so much.

Christen, 44: I'll miss them like crazy.

Brian, 43: I think that I could become very depressed or even get sick again, and maybe even wind up going back to the hospital.

Jay, 56: There was no change other than psychological—everything else remained the same.

Rachel, 44: My mother died when I was a teenager. Because my mother was my major support system at that time, I was greatly lonely at the time. Also, my development as a young lady was neglected because she was not there to help me learn such things. Since then my father has become a major source of support emotionally. I will suffer greatly when he dies.

Liana, 50: I'm glad that my mother is no longer around to listen to my schizophrenia.

Have you ever been married (how long)? Divorced? How did or does your mental illness affect your marriage?

Jade, 43: Fifteen years marriage—divorced seven because of my mental illness.

Danny Green, 46: Yes, I was married for two years. Not a great amount, although it did provide my wife an alibi for desertion.

Brunhilda, 44: I've been dating my boyfriend for 16 years. We cannot get married because he doesn't make enough money to pay for himself, let alone to pay my medical bills.

Will, 38: Never married. Mental illness would only affect my marriage if my kids got sick, hopefully making it stronger. I would not marry a woman who could not see what mental illness contributes to the genius, beauty, and creative nature of my mind.

> A study in 1989 places the single to married ratio worldwide for schizophrenics at 7.7:1 for men and 4.5:1 for women (Noll 264), as opposed to the U.S. general population in which 52% of men are married and 43% of women (2004 data from www.census.gov).

Harriet, 43: Married four years. Divorced 1998. Common-law marriage (now). Very happy.

Ozzie, 46: My wife divorced me because of my mental illness. But we got back together two years after hospitalization and Caramore. *(Editors' note: Caramore is a Vocational Rehabilitation program in Chapel Hill.)*

Jill, 27: I had a common-law marriage that didn't work out. I don't want to talk about that any more. Now I am engaged to someone I really care about who also has mental illness.

Aileen, 54: Divorced—my disorder made my married life more difficult, and I heard my husband say things he didn't say. I acted inappropriately.

Black Madonna, 36: I have been married for 10 happy years now—with lots of ups and downs. We have money issues because I like to spend lots of money.

Christen, 44: I've been married twice. The first time was only a year. This time it's right. We've been married for 25 years.

Brian, 43: I have never been married. Probably because I have the illness.

Jay, 56: Yes, I was married for six years. I am now divorced. The divorce occurred when I became ill.

Do you currently have a significant other? For how long? Do you have children? What ages?

Socrates, 43: Within the last month, I have begun a relationship with a wonderful woman. We have much in common and already love each other deeply. My last relationship was five years ago, and it was stressful and complicated.

Danny Green, 46: Yes, my son is eight years old.

Brunhilda, 44: I do not have children because I do not think I'm competent enough or have enough money to raise them properly. In addition to this, sometimes I wonder what their genetic make-up would be.

Will, 38: Solo and celibate for almost a decade. I do not think I have any children.

Jane, 53: My only "significant other" is the Lord. I have no children.

Barnaby, 23: I don't have a girlfriend or kids.

Harriet, 43: Currently married. No children, one doggie.

Ozzie, 46: No children. I am living with my ex-wife.

Jill, 27: Yes, about a year. No children.

Aileen, 54: I have had a significant other for 16 years. I have four children from two marriages, ages 35, 34, 22, and 20.

Black Madonna, 36: No children. I lost a baby full-term to still birth, nine years ago on June 2nd.

Christen, 44: One son, 27 years old.

Jay, 56: No. I have a son, 34 years old.

Is your family supportive? Explain why or why not. Who in your family supports you the most?

Jade, 43: Extremely. My mother and father and my cousins in the Midwest have all helped me a great deal.

Socrates, 43: My family is very supportive. My greatest support comes from my father and brother, who have grown to accept my illness. They have seen me in dire circumstances and now are amazed at the healing I have experienced. Both take a great interest in my life and support me emotionally. My brother has also sparked motivation for my writing.

Adam, 28: No, kind of. Nobody.

Danny Green, 46: Yes, they keep in touch. My sister Julia is most supportive.

Brunhilda, 44: My family is very supportive. One of my sisters is a physician, one majored in psychology, and my other sister and brother are well-educated. My mother is the most supportive of the family. She is very active in the mental health community and is constantly learning more about mental illness.

Zelda, 48: Most of my family takes a hands-off attitude. I tried to engage them—it didn't work. My mother, though, is my main source of support.

Will, 38: Mother and siblings support me how it matters most—with love and friendship. I think my father is just pleased and agog that I have come so far. I have enjoyed silencing those who doubted simply with significant life progress.

Jane, 53: My family is very much in favor of my taking medicine. In that sense, it is very supportive. It also is in favor of my studying and finding work. Sometimes, relatives have tried to impose their own priorities in my life, to which I have reacted rather negatively. Since I was diagnosed with the major mental illness, these relatives have been more understanding than they formerly were.

Barnaby, 23: I really don't confide in my family when it comes to symptoms. I don't think they could bear it if they knew—but maybe that says more about me than about them. I wouldn't be able to handle the questions and concern.

Harriet, 43: Very supportive. My father is very supportive emotionally and financially.

Ozzie, 46: Yes, my wife is very supportive. I don't talk to the rest of my family much.

> Research on family psychoeducation indicates that those program that last nine months to a year, with regular family participation, can reduce hospitalization rates up to 50% (mentalhealth.samhsa.gov).

Larry, 46: For a long time it was my grandmother who never judged me and provided a place to come. My father and I are probably closer than ever. My mother and I have had to mend some fences, but our love is stronger than in the past.

Jill, 27: Yes—mother and father and grandma do everything in their power to be there for me when I need them, and I am grateful.

Aileen, 54: My family is supportive. My partner and sister support me the most.

Black Madonna, 36: Yes, because they believe in learning all they can about mental illness. My husband is the most supportive.

Christen, 44: My husband, mom, and dad all give me support.

Brian, 43: Yes, my family is supportive. Especially my sister. And lately even my father. Mostly my older sister is still very loving and supportive.

Jay, 56: Yes, I come from a medical family—all are supportive.

Liana, 50: Yes, my brother says I can get diet pills. My brother is my payee.

How important to you are friendships with other people who have mental illness? Do you prefer these friendships to ones with others without mental illness?

Jade, 43: It is very important to have friends you can share "war" stories with. I take my friends one person at a time. Everybody has a story to tell.

Socrates, 43: My friendships with other people with mental illness are very important to me, especially since my nearest family members are 500 miles away. I feel a bond with them, and I know our sharing of experiences helps heal both them and me. I have several friends who do not have mental illness, and these are strong relationships, but I would say that I prefer those relationships with people who have mental illness because we have common experiences and I feel at ease to be myself with them.

Adam, 28: Very important. Learned a lot. No difference.

Danny Green, 46: Very important, but I do not necessarily value relationships with consumers over others.

Brunhilda, 44: I prize my relationships with other consumers. We can compare our experiences, and they seem to judge me less. I wish I could have more meaningful experiences and interactions with others without mental illness, with them treating me as they do other normal friends. That doesn't happen to me.

Zelda, 48: Crucial.

Will, 38: Very. I enjoy any genuine relationships, whatever the context: friends, colleagues, family.

Jane, 53: I am glad to be friends with other people who have mental illness. I am friends with my aunt by marriage and with many members at the clubhouse. We seem to make friends easily. Nevertheless, I do not want my friendships to be restricted to mentally ill people, and I really cherish my relationships with my family members and with other mentally healthy people for that reason.

Barnaby, 23: Maybe I do prefer friendships with others who are mentally ill. There is no front or façade. I don't have to pretend. I can just be me. There's a whole new level of friendship when you and your friend both have problems.

Harriet, 43: The friendships are very important and deep with mental illness.

Ozzie, 46: I have a lot of friends at work. I associate with my wife's friends who have mental illness.

Larry, 46: It is natural to interact with others who have similar problems or interests.

Jill, 27: I can't begin to say how important. Most of my friends have some sort of mental illness, but I can't say which I prefer.

Aileen, 54: Very important—both are good.

Black Madonna, 36: They are very important to me—I prefer friendships with people with mental illness because they tend to be genuine and true.

Christen, 44: I prefer friends with mental illness because they're special people and have similar lives.

Brian, 43: My relationships with other people who have the illness are very important because we can understand and support each other. Also, relationships with clubhouse staff are very important.

Jay, 56: Very important, and as important as those without.

Liana, 50: They are important because most of them are educated.

When you think of the people who are (or were) most helpful to you, what kind of things do they have in common?

Jade, 43: Compassion—they see beyond the illness.

Socrates, 43: I would say that the people that have helped me the most share the common attribute of non-judgmental love. They do not view me as "abnormal," but as someone who has a disability and yet has something to contribute.

Adam, 28: Compassion.

Danny Green, 46: Education and compassion.

Brunhilda, 44: They all have some of these assets:
- They have a lifestyle of helping others on a regular basis.
- They're well educated.
- They possess empathy of others, not just me.
- They listen and try to understand.
- They're genuinely interested in people.
- They respect others as individuals.
- They don't dwell on assumptions and stigma.

Will, 38: Few, in fact only one, had faith in my recovery. He is my best friend from college. Everyone else was convinced over time.

Jane, 53: The people most helpful to me usually have faith in Jesus Christ in common. I must specifically point out that my father helps me. He has expertise in legal matters and supervises my expenditures and records.

Barnaby, 23: They cared and took the time to try and understand what was going on and how I felt.

Harriet, 43: Psychiatrists—for 24 years treated me very well.

Ozzie, 46: I think they have a deep compassion for one another.

Larry, 46: Employment, having a mental illness, family.

Jill, 27: They are all very supportive and all very intelligent.

Aileen, 54: They seem to be naturally supportive.

Black Madonna, 36: Empathy, caring, and concerned people.

Christen, 44: My past preacher was most understanding because he understood and took time with people.

Brian, 43: They are usually people who do not succumb to the stigma associated with mental illness and are positive in their thinking about people who have mental illness.

Jay, 56: Women, MSW.

Rachel, 44: They are open-minded, intelligent, non-judgmental, and compassionate.

Liana, 50: My social worker has relatives from the Finger Lakes region like I do. I have Italian relatives like a club house member. He and I like to talk about our ancestry.

How do your spiritual/religious beliefs affect how you view your illness?

Jade, 43: I believe God has a special reason and place for the mentally ill. Our illness draws us closer.

Socrates, 43: My spiritual beliefs are the foundation of how I view my illness and are the greatest contributor to my healing. I have a deep and intimate relationship with God and have his constant companionship and support. I believe that there is a strong spiritual component to mental illness that affects physical, psychological, and emotional well-being. I know that I cannot prove God's existence to anyone, but I feel that God can prove himself to anyone.

Danny Green, 46: God should never be blamed for ill health. God is in healing.

Will, 38: My spirituality, mind, and body—along with any label that comes my way—have all been rolled into one over time. My commitment to wellness has made me the man I am today.

Jane, 53: I hope for a cure. When I was on Geodon, it did not work for me; but I clung to my faith in Jesus Christ and His message that I was forgiven, and I did not have a nervous breakdown, even when I was getting so little sleep that the psychiatrist had to prescribe Am-

> In a recent study, 30% of persons with schizophrenia reported "an increase in their religiousness after the onset of their illness" (Torrey 363).

bien for temporary help. I know that disobedience has led to the gravity of my illness, but I also hope that the Lord will heal me soon. The whole experience has impressed me that I need to obey the Lord more than I have done in the past.

Barnaby, 23: I used to think my illness was a form of demon possession. Actually, for a while, I stopped taking my meds thinking I needed spiritual cure, not a physiological one. Now I think maybe they're one and the same. I do believe that the voices are demons, but for some reason, I hesitate to call it possession.

Harriet, 43: My psychiatrist does not believe in God but says it is in my best interest to believe in God.

Larry, 46: Many times they create confusion and an unhealthy thought process.

Black Madonna, 36: One day I will be healed completely from my illness. One day I will not have to take meds.

Christen, 44: It's hard. My religion gives me hope. I pray a lot, maybe too much.

Brian, 43: I view mental illness as one of the very many forms of suffering in the world and that there is a compassionate God who wishes to remove that suffering.

Rachel, 44: Because of my spiritual beliefs, I am more patient and accepting of my illness and my difficulties.

Liana, 50: I have faith in God.

In what ways have your spiritual/religious beliefs been an asset or a hindrance to your health?

Jade, 43: They have helped give me a sense of purpose, which is an asset to my health.

Socrates, 43: I would say that my spiritual beliefs have been both an asset and a factor in my illness. My focus on the spiritual has led to many spiritual battles which have been the primary focus of my psychosis. But my faith has also sustained me in these tough experiences and been the source of much healing.

Zelda, 48: I am not a victim.

Will, 38: Pardon me, but religion f***s everything up. Spirituality erases the barriers and eliminates the distance that religious practices impose on humanity. Managing a once-intractable mind has given birth to a spirit and hunger for life that I never otherwise would have had.

Jane, 53: Once I thought that the Lord was healing me, but I needed to wait for His message of forgiveness to get through to me. When it comes in fullness, God willing, this healing will be not superficial, but deep.

Barnaby, 23: Religion gave me a place to start and something to hang on to when things were bad. I also could comfort myself when the demons were really bothering me. I'd pray to God and Jesus to help.

Harriet, 43: I have been angry at God, but I believe that he is a compassionate God.

Aileen, 54: Praying helps.

Black Madonna, 36: It has helped me to have a balance. Prayer has centered me. It has helped me to be calm.

> Fifty percent of people with schizophrenia experience religious delusions (Torrey 363), which are classified as grandiose delusions. Individuals with schizophrenia commonly believe they are God, Jesus Christ, or a prophet (Noll 334). The onset of illness is commonly at a time when philosophical beliefs are being formed. Auditory hallucinations can reinforce grandiose delusions (Torrey 363).

Christen, 44: Praying too much keeps me from doing other things.

Brian, 43: In some ways it is helpful, but it can also be difficult if other people who are religious are judgmental and stigmatizing.

Jay, 56: An asset for they help me be optimistic and hopeful.

Liana, 50: My minister brought my luggage to me even though he knew I was suffering.

Elaborations...

Brunhilda, 44: My older sister, the doctor, and my little sister both had children in the same time period. Shortly after each of their children was born, they were into who in the family their children most looked like (as new parents often do). They were most bothered by genetic similarities between their children and those that only the children's aunt (me) possess. I knew what they were trying to determine, and I never said a word. Ultimately, if their children received "bad genes," I am not to blame. It would be impossible to be my fault.

These kids are terrific. Sometimes I wonder how they will treat me when they're older and find out I'm "crazy." Surely they'll find out before they're old enough or educated enough to understand mental illness. I'm just so apprehensive about my future role of the "crazy aunt."

It's like my artwork. My niece goes around telling people her aunt is an artist, and she wants to be a good artist like her aunt. How old will she be when she realizes her aunt's artwork isn't that great? Surely, the stigma of having a crazy aunt will overshadow any value as an artist.

Jane, 53: Nearly every night I have what I call a "pill ceremony," during which I show each of my parents the pill I have to take that night. Then I take the pill, and they can watch me if they'd like. Sometimes my father forgets whether or not he has seen the pill, and if it weren't for my mother remembering she saw it, I'd really be in a bad situation. My father has an awful temper, and he gets very uptight when he gets some notion that I have not taken my pill at the proper time.
Once I went on a little vacation with my mother. Each night of the vacation, I faithfully showed her my pill for the night and took it. When I got back, my father asked me if I had ever taken a pill while I was away. I was so disgusted and angry at him that I didn't even bother to answer. Perhaps mother told him what had happened—I just turned aside and held my temper.

Barnaby, 23: I think a lot of people's reaction to someone who is sick is to give them a wide berth and avoid them or let them be. But I think that socialization is extremely important to someone who is ill. Having spent some two years in practical isolation, I can tell you that if you have schizophrenia or schizoaffective disorder, you need more people than someone who is well.

Liana, 50: I have been feeling despair about the way I look. The female staff are all attractive. I recently had my front tooth repaired, which was chipped. I now feel "born to win"—the name of one of my favorite books. Right now I just need to consume less calories.

Community Living

Insanity – a perfectly rational adjustment to an insane world.

– R. D. Laing

A Thousand Decembers

– Samantha Bierman

Stronger than love
deeper than spiritual
nothing short of
a soul-to-soul miracle.
I've seen it before
but only in pictures
with decadent curtains
and chandelier fixtures,
passion and fever
burning like embers
flying through blue skies
for a thousand Decembers.
I once wandered aimlessly
scared to go forward
now I have a target
that's worth walking toward
and even if tragedy
comes overnight
I'll feel your electricity
charging my light
and if you love someone better
I'll stand and fight

I'll back you up always
when your cause is right
'cause we're stronger than love
deeper than spiritual
and nothing short of
a soul-to-soul miracle.

What poses the most difficult day-to-day living situation for you?

Jade, 43: Managing money, finances.

Socrates, 43: Work sometimes poses difficulties with anxiety and paranoia (on bad days). On good days, I have a great time.

Adam, 28: Remembering to take my medicine.

Danny Green, 46: Nothing outward, just the malfunctions of my brain.

Brunhilda, 44: I hate grocery shopping the most. It is always crowded, and the people shopping there are almost always rude. Now I go to the Super Walmart at 6:00 Sunday mornings. I go as little as possible.

Zelda, 48: The entire transportation situation is problematic.

Will, 38: Working all week leaves time on the weekend only for laundry and sleep, or so it seems. Shopping with good coupons before EBT* was pretty humbling, I must say. *(*Editors' note: EBT was previously known as food stamps.)*

Jane, 53: Driving is the most difficult and something about which I pray a lot. There are so many tall plants that grow in my neighborhood that visibility can be sadly weakened.

Barnaby, 23: I have the most trouble paying attention at school and doing schoolwork that isn't due the next day. I keep thinking I'll sit and quietly read the necessary material, but that doesn't happen very often.

Harriet, 43: Bathing.

Larry, 46: Eating healthy.

Jill, 27: Cleaning.

Aileen, 54: Time alone.

Black Madonna, 36: Just getting out of bed has been a difficult situation in the past. But working and holding a job tends to be most difficult.

Christen, 44: I don't like grocery shopping because it takes so long and there are always so many people.

> Life events and daily hassles are the two categories of life which cause people stress. Life events are stressful to everyone. To people with schizophrenia, simple daily hassles (including personal hygiene, household chores, transportation, shopping, errands, and routing medical appointments) may be experienced as extremely stressful, sometimes more even than life events (Mueser and Gingrich 156).

Brian, 43: The hardest part of my day is getting out of bed in the morning due to the sedative effect of my medication.

Jay, 56: Being away from the nursing home.

Rachel, 44: Working is almost impossible because of interpersonal difficulties. I prefer not to work because it allows me to participate in other activities that are more important to me. Bus riding is difficult because everything takes three times as long. Shopping is a pleasure and an addiction.

Liana, 50: I received a new pair of scales for my birthday and gained five pounds. I work an hour a day in the club house, and sometimes I wonder if the other employees know it's a man's job.

Have you ever been in legal trouble due to your illness or faulty perception? What happened?

Jade, 43: I've been picked up by the police and taken to hospitals, but never charged in the courts.

> Twenty-four percent of state prison inmates and 21% of local jail inmates have had a recent mental illness (Uninsured and Costs 8).

Socrates, 43: I have had only one problematic interaction with the law. I was arrested for vagrancy when I was homeless and entered a department store to seek warmth and a place to rest. The police eventually took me to a hospital.

Brunhilda, 44: No, knock wood. I understand how it can happen to the mentally ill, especially charges of loitering and trespassing.

Will, 38: Not to my knowledge. I have never been charged with or convicted of any crime. No matter what I have imagined doing, whether from crazy or just stupid, I now just walk the straight and narrow. Woe is me…

Jane, 53: Thank God I've avoided trouble with the law. The hospital lawyer has seen me a couple of times, but nothing significant happened as a result.

Ozzie, 46: Yes, I got two misdemeanors when I was ill.

> One thousand homicides a year are attributed to schizophrenia and bipolar disorder. There is a 50% reduction in violence after treatment (www.psychlaws. org/GeneralResources/Fact1.htm).

Larry, 46: Hospitalized for stealing.

Liana, 50: I lost my mother in January of 1979, and the police handcuffed me.

What problems have you encountered in various living situations? Have you ever experienced illegal discrimination during or after finding a housing situation?

What happened?

Socrates, 43: I have had only one housing dilemma. After a psychotic break I found myself homeless. After several hospitalizations in another state, I returned home to my roommate, and he had me evicted (I was not on the lease). Once again, I was homeless.

Brunhilda, 44: There was a situation where someone wouldn't rent to my boyfriend and me. I don't know if it was legal or not. I do know that cohabitation is illegal in North Carolina. Which is the worse sin, cohabitation or being one of the worst slum lords I've come across?

> Most crimes against those with a psychiatric illness are not reported, from the stealing of disability checks to rape and murder (www.psychlaws.org/GeneralResources/Fact1.htm).

Zelda, 48: Thank goodness this has never happened.

Will, 38: No, quite the contrary, I enjoyed almost a decade in safe, decent, affordable government housing and now look forward to ownership of real property.

Jane, 53: Cleaning my room seems to be a perpetual problem. I am not a particularly neat person. I have lived with my parents for years, and they are very patient with me about this. Once I rented a room from an old lady, now deceased, who lived near my family. She wanted to do things together more often than I found I could. I have never experienced illegal discrimination concerning a housing situation.

Harriet, 43: Bad roommates.

Ozzie, 46: At Dorothea Dix, my roommate would put lotion on his penis and masturbate when I was in the room.

Larry, 46: Early on, it was difficult staying in one place for an extended time.

Aileen, 54: Making or getting enough money to meet expenses.

Brian, 43: I have been near homelessness a couple of times. I have been "kicked out" of halfway houses and have had to rely on hospitals at times for shelter.

> The website www.schizophrenia.com has a number of articles on crime, poverty and mental illness. For example, the site states that one third of the estimated 600,000 homeless population suffers from an untreated psychiatric illness.

Rachel, 44: I have had lots of problems with neighbors not wanting me to be a neighbor.

Liana, 50: I was evicted from three attractive apartments in 1979 because I had two cats.

What percentage of your income do you spend on housing, and what type of housing do you have? Are you happy in this situation?

Jade, 43: I rent a lovely apartment. It is a third of my income. I am very happy with the situation.

Socrates, 43: I spend only one-sixth of my income on housing which allows me to sink more money into the never-ending abyss of car repairs. I am very happy with my housing situation—I live in a boarding house that was built in 1920.

Adam, 28: A third of my income goes to rent in my apartment.

Danny Green, 46: Thirty-five percent of my income goes to rent of my apartment.

Brunhilda, 44: I rent a house with my boyfriend, and my share of the rent is about 50% of my income. I would like to live in a nicer house, but you have to pay for what you get.

Zelda, 48: One half.

Will, 38: In government housing, 30%, which ranges from 0 to $700, depending on my employment and government benefits—SSI and Medicaid. I lost all income in graduate school, and I was housed for free for quite some time.

Jane, 53: I spend none of my income on housing because my parents let me stay with them for free. Sometimes I think I'd like to leave, but it depends on what the conflict is. I have been fairly happy with this situation of having my own room in my parents' house.

Harriet, 43: I rent my townhouse and spend a third of my Social Security check on rent.

Ozzie, 46: Yes, I'm happy. I spend $250 a month on rent, and $200 to $250 a month on utilities. I live with my ex-wife in a townhouse.

Larry, 46: One-third, yes, renting an apartment.

Jill, 27: Have my own house. About half my income. Yes, I am happy.

Aileen, 54: Twenty-five percent is spent on housing. I have a house-mate and we own the house together.

Black Madonna, 36: Seventy-five percent on housing—own home—no—I would like to buy another home—I need more space.

Christen, 44: I live with my husband, and we own the house.

Brian, 43: I spend about 30% of my annual income on rent, and I live in an apartment that is managed by the Mental Health Association, and my rent is on a sliding scale basis.

Jay, 56: I stay in a nursing home where all my money from SSDI goes to pay for my care. I get an allowance of $30 a month.

Rachel, 44: I am very happy with my living situation. I spend a third of my income on rent. I rent a very nice and very safe apartment in a great location.

Liana, 50: I have Section 8 housing.

If you live in a group home, or lived in one in the past, what were the benefits, and what were the challenges?

Socrates, 43: After being homeless, a non-profit organization housed me in a group home. I enjoyed this living situation a lot because of the support and comradeship of my fellow housemates who also had mental illness. Eventually I got a job and a place to live, but the group home helped me begin recovery.

Adam, 28: No benefits, no privacy.

Danny Green, 46: Avoiding the streets; lacking privacy.

Ozzie, 46: Worrying about your stuff being stolen and getting along with room-mates that had problems.

Larry, 46: Having numerous personalities getting along at one time.

> **Where We Live:**
> 6% Homeless in Shelters
> 6% Prisons and Jails
> 5% Hospitals
> 10% Nursing Homes
> 28% Live Independently
> 20% Supervised Housing
> 25% Live with Family Members
> (Torrey 409)

Brian, 43: I lived in two different group homes and one halfway house. The group homes were good for socialization and learning how to live independently in the community. The halfway house was completely useless.

Jay, 56: Getting my medical needs met.

Liana, 50: I lived in a rest home, and one of the benefits was that they allowed pets.

Elaborations...

Jane, 53: Actually, I do not know if this is an anecdote, but sometimes in my darkest moods, the psychiatric business seems like a sort of racket, the object of which is to make me and keep me dependent on pills. It even seemed that way before I started my appointments with UNC Hospital psychiatrists. I was very deeply upset when I was taking Trilafon, and I got so confused that I didn't remember the difference between left and right. As I said, fortunately, my mother was driving. I let the psychiatrists hear plenty about it after we got back to town! I used to have anxieties that the floors were not thick or strong enough to hold the weight of all us humans who had to be on them. Nevertheless, my most difficult anxieties have often seemed to come when someone else was driving.

When my father is driving us to a nearby city, I can get terribly anxious. So many drivers seem to speed and not to signal when they change lanes, that I keep in fairly constant, silent prayer. I also thank God that it is my father who is doing the driving. He has much more experience with highway traffic than I do, and his nerves seem steady.

When we had the snow storm in 2000, I was deeply thankful for all the times he did the driving; he has had much more experience with snow and ice than I have had, and we then had several health emergencies in the family. As for me, the Lord seems to keep me steady and free from panic when we are on the highway, but if it weren't for Him, I don't know what I would do.

Several times when mother and I drove to the beach, she wanted me to have the maps and to be a sort of navigator. She wanted to drive, and I was happy to let her. Nevertheless, when I was on Geodon, I nagged her all the way there. I don't know how she put up with me. My behavior was just awful. I prayed too, which outlet kept things from getting worse. I hated traveling at the speed with which we had to drive on the highway. Any time there was the slightest turn in the road, I would pray like mad that we would follow it and not crash through the barrier and wind up in a ditch or rammed into a tree. My mother is a very safe driver and does not deserve to be treated the way I treated her when I was on Geodon. I was grateful that she was driving when we were on the busy roads homeward in the afternoon traffic. She has driven beautifully, all the way to the beach and back, several times. She deserves better treatment from me. I hope that I will learn soon how not to be in such a dreadful state on the highways

Liana, 50: I received a pair of scales for my birthday and remember my brother saying, "You don't want scales." He might have been absolutely right because I gained five pounds since then. I am reminded of an article in Weight Watchers' about this lady who said, after she got on the scales, "Why are you looking at me like that?" and the lady with her said, "Because you just screamed."

Socrates, 43: I once had a psychotic break and fled in my car north. I ended up in another state and was stopped by a policeman for swerving in the road (as I hadn't slept in three or four days). I had a bag of medicine in my car, and when the policeman saw this, he brought me to a hospital. It was a private hospital, and since I had no insurance (and had not yet received disability), they sent me to a public institution after one week.

The psychiatric ward was full, so they put me in a forensic unit with psychiatric criminals. I stayed in this institution for about two weeks, after which I took the doctor to court and won my liberty. He was so incensed with me, he put me out on the street with no money, no way back to my car, and no medicine. I was left homeless in a place I did not even know.

I suffered extreme thirst, hunger, cold and psychosis until I found a hospital and was sent to another institution. After one month, I was put on a bus back to my hometown, and eventually hospitalized again.

A social worker at the hospital placed me with a non-profit organization that helps the mentally ill. I was given a job and a place to live, and they got me my disability. I now hold a job and live on my own. With governmental assistance and God's love, I have put my life back together.

Education and Employment

Imagination is more important than knowledge.

– Albert Einstein

To Hope

– Rhonda Allen

I will survive because I cry.
In hurt.
Repair.
In sleep.
Hope, pray I cry to heal so deep.

I will survive because I seek.
To touch.
Protect.
In speech.
Hope, pray I seek to heal so deep.

I survive to love.
Give up.
Get back…
Then grow
Learn to need…survive to know.

Survived I have.
Some tried…some died.
Not me.
I was, I will, I am… I'll be.

To hope I pray to die tonight.
That part of me of single sight.
Where lives only trouble, angst, and fright.
May God forgive me and send his light.

I'm in you and you're in me.
I was, I will, I am.
You see… We're we.
And God always sees.
Because of hope I grew to me.

Have you had difficulties in your education because of your illness? What was your greatest challenge?

Jade, 43: I was in the middle of my master's degree when it hit.

Socrates, 43: I had a precursor to my illness at 19 years old due to smoking marijuana laced with PCP (unbeknownst to me). I was healthy for eight years before it resurfaced and so I managed to complete my education.

Adam, 28: Yes, being suicidal, depression, delusions.

Danny Green, 46: Yes, there was always a flare-up. A brain disease will close down both intellectual and emotional pursuits. Reading, writing, taking notes, all suffer.

Brunhilda, 44: I almost had to change my major in college, which was art. I shook so badly from lithium, I could not participate in a drawing class. Erratic student hours did not help with being bipolar. I had a very rough time in college from trying to understand my mental illness, to attending early-morning classes. I was on so much medication, I had to hook my loud stereo on a timer to wake up.

Zelda, 48: This question is tough to answer—I got my diagnosis well after college.

Will, 38: Graduating from college was a neat trick, if not a miracle. In graduate school, years into my recovery, managing workload and stress was critical.

> 50% of students age 14 and up with mental illness quit high school. This is the highest drop-out rate of any disability group (Uninsured and Costs 8).

Jane, 53: I believe that my greatest educational difficulty was in figuring out what a sentence said when I was taking courses in ancient Greek.

Those people did not always have the same kind of syntax that we do. I think the greatest challenge in my general education was the loneliness and depression that I often felt. If not for them, I think I could have gotten higher grades than I did.

Barnaby, 23: I had to take a couple of years off of school because of my illness. Even after I came back, though, my symptoms kept me from learning new material and getting homework done; my illness kept me from doing well. Only now, after five years of illness, do I feel close to where I was before I got sick, with respect to how I'm doing in school.

Harriet, 43: I had great difficulty getting my B.A. degree. I was committed during exam week.

Larry, 46: Dropped out of college. Realizing I had an illness.

Jill, 27: Yes, in high school I was barely able to graduate because I went on a manic spree and would not attend classes.

Aileen, 54: Not being able to go back to school due to too much stress and also fear of losing my disability.

Black Madonna, 36: Yes! I am a slow learner – taking notes – math has been my greatest challenge.

Christen, 44: All through school I was a slow learner.

Brian, 43: Yes, I have had huge difficulty with my education due to my mental illness. I was in college when I first began to get sick and was completely unable to continue or to finish college, and I have never gone back.

Jay, 56: Anxiety in doing bio-lab work.

Rachel, 44: Inability to retain as much and to think as clearly. For a long time when the work became stressful I would become obsessed with something else and not attend to the project at hand.

Liana, 50: No difficulties in education, but I took an anthropology course in the fall of 1981 which was as difficult as a graduate course.

Have you retrained or re-schooled for a different type of work or career after facing limitations due to your mental illness?

Socrates, 43: After I was no longer able to teach, I went to nursing school for one year, and although I did well in school, I found that nursing would be too stressful for me to handle, and dropped out of the program in my final year.

> One in seven college students report difficulty at school due to mental illness (College Life 17).

Adam, 28: Caramore grounds crew and cleaning crew.

Danny Green, 46: Yes, I've studied forestry, offset printing, and child care.

Brunhilda, 44: I could not handle white-collar jobs. I was too paranoid of internal politics as well as unable to deal with the people. I re-schooled in horticulture (an AAS degree). Blue-collar jobs, all you have to do is work hard, get the job done, and that's all that matters.

Will, 38: Nope. I plan to return for another graduate degree some day. Glutton for punishment.

Jane, 53: Yes. I have trained in computer use after finding out that I had schizoaffective disorder.

Barnaby, 23: There are some classes I'd like to take, but until now, I haven't felt up to it.

Ozzie, 46: Yes, now I'm a bagger at Harris Teeter, and I used to work in construction, which was very hard work.

Jill, 27: I am currently at a community college working on a certification. I hope it works out!

Aileen, 54: Not so far, although I have had to have additional support at work.

Liana, 50: I changed my major for the third time in 1981. I was glad I did—I was skinny but also depressed because someone was following me. One wish did come true however—I was a skinny co-ed.

> Vocational Rehabilitation Services is a state agency that assists disabled individuals with education and employment issues. They test for interests and abilities and help develop work skills. After helping with job placement, job coaching is available (Smith 11).

Have you worked for pay since you were diagnosed with mental illness? Are you currently working? What type of work?

Jade, 43: No. I volunteer at the thrift shop.

Socrates, 43: I currently work part-time helping manage a used-book store. I have flexibility in my schedule, and though working with the public is sometimes difficult for me, much of my time is spent sorting, pricing, stocking, and keeping inventory.

Adam, 28: Yes. No.

Danny Green, 46: Yes, for 30 years. No.

Brunhilda, 44: I have been out of work for three years. Previously, I had a wonderful part-time job on the grounds of a museum, landscaping and in the greenhouses. Everyone always commented on how hard I worked.

Zelda, 48: No—SSI.

Will, 38: Full-time for almost two years as a trained professional, astoundingly enough. I'm definitely on the treadmill with lofty goals in my career and life.

> "The annual economic, indirect cost for mental illness is estimated at $79 billion, $69 billion is from loss of productivity" (Uninsured and Costs 8).

Jane, 53: I have worked in at least one temporary job for pay, after being diagnosed. I am currently studying, not working for pay.

Barnaby, 23: I used to give a few tennis lessons here and there. I don't work now.

Harriet, 43: Yes, retail, various entry-level jobs. No.

Ozzie, 46: Yes, I work as a bagger.

> According to the U.S. Census Bureau, the unemployment rate for people with disabilities is 44.2%, almost 10 times the national unemployment rate (Drummond B4B).

Larry, 46: Yes, employed in a clubhouse program.

Jill, 27: For one month at WalMart.

Aileen, 54: I work for pay now. I do office work.

Black Madonna, 36: I have worked three transitional-employment jobs through Club Nova. I once worked at the Orange County public library for six months. I worked at the Mental Health Association for one year. I worked a couple of weeks at the YMCA.

Christen, 44: I worked at a cafeteria for two years, but that was 10 years ago.

Brian, 43: Yes, I have worked several different types of jobs and currently am working in a van driving job for the clubhouse.

Liana, 50: I worked in 1979 at a fast food restaurant in Pennsylvania. I also worked at the university mail room in 2004-2005. I'm currently working an hour a day, five days a week.

Have you ever told a boss you had mental illness? Did it work out?

Socrates, 43: After two years working part-time, I told my boss about my illness. I had already proven my reliability so he had no problem with it.

Brunhilda, 44: At my last job, my boss knew I had mental illness when he hired me. Once, I had failed a drug trial, was hallucinating, not eating, and not sleeping. They gave me two weeks off. That has never happened to me—usually they just fire me.

Will, 38: Yep. These days my strengths eclipse my weaknesses, or so I choose to believe. Each day that passes, I become more successful at using my vulnerabilities to my advantage, simply by staying true to myself.

Jane, 53: When I did temporary work, the boss knew I had mental illness. She mistreated me in no way.

Barnaby, 23: I had worked for my dad. He already knew.

Harriet, 43: Yes. I got fired after five years.

Ozzie, 46: No, I never did. I'm afraid they might fire me if they found out.

> The Equal Employment Opportunity Commission (EEOC) monitors employment practices and assists people with disabilities to ensure that they are not victims of unfair employment practices.

Larry, 46: Yes, they appreciated my honesty and gave me a job I had for 33 months.

Aileen, 54: Yes, I told her at the interview for the job. My counselor was one of my references and advocated for me.

Black Madonna, 36: Yes. No it didn't—they fired me.

Christen, 44: My boss at the cafeteria knew. It may have helped, I don't know.

Brian, 43: No, but the people I work for at the clubhouse know me and know that I have a mental illness.

Rachel, 44: I tend not to tell anyone that I deal with professionally (school, work, volunteer positions) because I have found that my diagnosis tends to cause people to underestimate me.

Have you ever faced stigma at work? What happened? How did you handle it?

Socrates, 43: I have dealt with some stigma at work, not so much in words but posture. Whispers behind my back, condescension, and the like. At first it frustrated me, but I just loved my coworkers to death, and they gradually accepted me and even grew to like me.

Brunhilda, 44: When I experience stigma at work, it's usually from coworkers. I've had a lot of jobs that don't require much education.

Uneducated people seem to possess more stigma. All you can do about stigma is try to prove their negative assumptions wrong.

Will, 38: Nope. People have troubled me, but I take a certain amount of pleasure in eventually proving people wrong.

Jane, 53: At first, the other workers seemed not to know quite how to treat me and were a little reserved. Nevertheless, when they observed me working steadily and not having all kinds of problems with what I was doing, they seemed to gradually get over their qualms or fears and to treat me like just another one of the office personnel.

Barnaby, 23: No stigma—I worked for my father.

Harriet, 43: Yes. I was resentful. I responded by getting a disability check.

Ozzie, 46: Sometimes it gets stressful when it is really busy. I try to go in the bathroom to get away from the stress, or get a drink of water.

Larry, 46: Only the stigma I placed on myself, which deteriorated my employment.

Black Madonna, 36: Yes! When my employer found out I had been in a mental hospital, they fired me from my child-care job.

Brian, 43: I have never worked anywhere where they knew about my illness, except for the clubhouse.

Liana, 50: I was followed by what is known as the body snatchers. I threw a temper tantrum, but no one heard it.

Do you think the side effects of your medication affect your ability to work? How so?

Jade, 43: Absolutely. I get tired. I get confused. I can only handle 2-3 hours a day.

Socrates, 43: In years past, medication definitely impeded my ability to work, primarily intense fatigue and sleepiness due to side effects. I also had tremors which made waiting tables difficult. But my present medication does not interfere with my current work.

Adam, 28: Yes, it slows me down.

Danny Green, 46: No, my disease does.

Brunhilda, 44: There are certain side effects I must be careful with in my profession. I get dizzy and pass out when I'm in hot sun or get up too fast. I have several skin conditions which are side effects that working outdoors makes them worse. I sunburn easily and have to walk/drive to go to the bathroom frequently. All in a day's work...

Zelda, 48: I don't know if I can work.

Will, 38: I need a lot of sleep when off the clock. My life is exhausting.

Jane, 53: I do not like being forgetful. Every once in a while, I need someone to repeat what he just said. I don't like that, and neither does the other person. Otherwise, I don't seem to have any problems doing work.

> According to one study of schizophrenia, 73% of people polled were not employed, 14.5% were competitively employed, and 12.6% were employed in non-competitive environments (ajp.psychiatryonline.org).

Barnaby, 23: For a long, long time my medication made me so tired I couldn't do anything. After some adjustments and a tolerance to the drowsiness, the meds don't affect me so strongly any more.

Harriet, 43: No—had to have a lot of water because of my dry mouth. I was penalized for using the bathroom too often.

Jill, 27: Yes, they wanted me to do physical labor, such as climbing ladders, and I felt dizzy and I just couldn't do it.

Aileen, 54: Not now, but before I was so sleepy I could hardly work.

Christen, 44: My main problem is being so tired I can't do anything.

Brian, 43: Yes, because I have trouble getting up in the morning due to the sedative effect of my medication.

Rachel, 44: Mostly by causing sleepiness.

Liana, 50: Someone told me when you were taking the drug, you didn't smile.

Have you ever experienced anxiety, paranoia, delusions or hallucinations at work? How did you cope?

Socrates, 43: I have experienced both anxiety and paranoia. To deal with the anxiety, I pray and try to calm my emotion, using biofeedback. When the paranoia comes, I tell myself that my thoughts are irrational and try to think of something positive.

Adam, 28: Yes, all of them. I didn't.

Brunhilda, 44: I'm constantly paranoid at any job I do. This definitely increases my anxiety level.

Will, 38: Not really. Some mild hypomanic and delusional thinking when I switched from Zyprexa to Abilify, but I was prepared by my doctor and anticipated this, and the cross-taper was handled successfully.

Jane, 53: I have sometimes been very careful at work about what I said. I would say that sometimes I have experienced anxiety at work. I prayed about it and went on doing what I thought was the best I could.

Barnaby, 23: I've experienced these things at school in class. I had a lot of trouble thinking people could hear my thoughts. It's nerve-wracking to monitor every thought that goes through your head and then I'd try not to think certain things for fear people could hear and would judge me crazy or stupid or just a big jerk. Of course, when you're worried about all that, you're not learning.

Harriet, 43: Yes. Medication.

Ozzie, 46: Sometimes I experience anxiety. I try to slow down and relax.

Larry, 46: Yes, the best I could until the situation deteriorated itself.

Jill, 27: Yes, I quit.

Aileen, 54: I have anxiety at work. I am on a medication to help. I take breaks. I just keep trying.

Christen, 44: No but I haven't worked in a very long time.

Brian, 43: Yes, I have had paranoia and delusions while working, and I mainly coped by not telling anyone and just trying to "stick it out."

Jay, 56: Yes, I tried to stay busy but eventually was dismissed.

Liana, 50: Once in 1976 I thought that "thanks" meant "T-Hanks." Another time a manager was talking about the "Electric Chainsaw Massacre."

Elaborations...

Brunhilda, 44: The older I get, regardless of how much I've recovered, it becomes harder and harder to find suitable employment. I re-schooled at a community college in a different field a few years ago. I prefer being in the blue-collar labor force, instead of undergoing the paranoia in white-collar jobs. Vocational Rehabilitation helped me find my wonderful current job (which is only seasonal and part-time). It took a long time to find.

For most individuals with schizophrenia, recovery is a long process. Not only does work help them build discipline, which they can use in other areas of their life, it builds self-esteem and provides them with another larger purpose. Beneficial work should be part of the recovery process when the individual is at a certain stage.

I've known clubhouse members who have had as many as six TE (Transitional Employment) jobs. Why is this necessary? Over the years I've only known one person whose TE job became permanent. I do not have a solution for this obvious dilemma. Should the clubhouse change its focus? Could they seek employers to hire the best of these individuals after their TE period? Should they work in conjunction with VR?

What I do know is that there should be different and more government work incentives. Part-time work should be a reward and a chance to live better financially. Also, being able to work more hours makes you more valuable and hirable to the employer.

I understand fully that the government's goal is ultimately that we to return back to work and be self-supporting. People recover from this illness gradually, and few can handle the jump from very part-time (most work 10-16 hours) straight to a full-time job (just about the only kind that will provide insurance). The only ones I've known to successfully do this were almost fully recovered, went to graduate school, and obtained their jobs shortly thereafter. It took them years of recovery and perseverance to get there.

Larry, 46: Concerning stigma on the job, my eventual supervisor said he chose me over six other applicants because I had been honest with him about my gap-filled employment and mental illness. I went on to work for 33 months with him—not always smooth, but successful for me.

Danny Green, 46: It was intramural track day at my high school, and I broke my arm. Flush with my win in the long-jump, I, like Icarus in the Greek myth, entered the high-jump, and my wings just plain melted. Having never mastered the Fosbury Flop, I clipped the bar on my third attempt at six feet and landed squarely on my right arm. Directly, I went into shock. Just as my classmates, with their innate compassion over-powered by their morbid curiosity, I too looked upon my right arm's second elbow with detached fascination.

This break tagged me in the merry month of May in my final successful term of education. I was 15. That summer found me in the glorious beauty of the George Washington National Forest, Lee Ranger District, Virginia. Working with my cast up to my right shoulder, I truly enjoyed the work, the baloney sandwiches, and the comaraderie of the Youth Conservation Corps. We maintained and blazed trails, fought off seven rattle snakes, canoed the Shenandoah River, and went caving along the West Virginia border.

In my first full brush with the realm of disability, the YCC blazed a Lions' Club trail for the blind, with signs in Braille and rocks to augment the roar of a waterfall on an adjacent stream. There was always something that compelled me to imagine a life without sight, without sound, and without walking. Also I could picture the drumbeat of death approaching us all.

The greatest spectacle of my YCC summer came on our hike up Kennedy Peak, thanks to God's blessing of mobility. The blessing of sight allowed us to witness the sheer glory of this perch! Its vista of Fort Valley (the valley within the valley) in the cleft of the Massanutten Mountain range, Passage Creek, and both north and south forks of the Shenandoah River overwhelmed us. As I was a straggler on this hike, I was too late to claim a spot in the shelter atop Kennedy Peak.

So three of us slept overnight in a cold July mountain rain on the roof of the shelter—the observation deck. There was a joke below in the dry shelter that the cast on my right arm would liquefy in the rain and trickle through the planks above! The following morning some other hikers shared some hot tea we made from surrounding sassafras roots at sunrise. We had a great time!

At the end of that summer, as my employment with the YCC was winding to a close, I felt the onslaught of impending doom. Although only 15, the clinical depression for which I would pay all my life since had revealed its viper's tongue. It was all very hard to tell.

My studies suffered greatly throughout the next academic year. Although I fancied myself good at language, my English course wound up in mutual hostility between my teacher and me. I hit the wall in pre-calculus. My chemistry teacher (who had a PhD in education and a master's in chemistry) labored valiantly but in vain. Latin and French went somewhat better, and my government teacher was brilliant.

Yet all the while I knew something was desperately wrong. There was a grave, gigantic but vague nothingness devouring all my nights and days. My brain had shut down like a diabolical mousetrap. This closed off both intellectual and social pursuits. My world had undergone an eclipse. Furthermore, I could not articulate the toll of the total damage. The undiagnosed brain disease progresses in its insidious, unchecked and malignant course, robbing the patient of the very voice to cry, "Help!"

With the money I'd earned for the summer job with the YCC, I purchased driver's education, 20 Beatles albums, and (at the insistence of my parents), a set of headphones. The next summer produced a number of abortive tries at conforming to the world around me. I scuttled both a job at the county public library and the drive for wheels. This summer also saw my first contact with what was then the scourge of the earth: The Psychiatric Profession.

Health & Substance Use and Abuse

When you stop drinking, you have to deal with this marvelous personality that started you drinking in the first place.

— Jimmy Breslin

Broken

– Mark Hutchinson

Shy and introspective
Lives in a dreamworld.
Picked upon.
No common sense,
The town fool.
He drinks away the pain,
He tries hard,
He dreams of success.
Suddenly, he stops fighting,
he is broken.

A new world.
Now he can only dream,
he rarely speaks,
dreaming of what might have been.
Life has been hard.

He lives for years.
Stuck in a capsule,
mind young,
yet hair graying.

Finally someone befriends him.
She loves him.

He can see for the first time.
He has been through a lot.
He is wise,
He is sane,
He is well.

How do you think exercise helps with the recovery process? What kind of exercise, if any, do you like to do?

Jade, 43: Definitely—I work out two hours a day—either swimming, biking, walking, or weight lifting.

Socrates, 43: Recently I have begun to swim, bike, weight-lift, and walk regularly. It helps my focus and gets those endorphins pumping. I especially like swimming.

Adam, 28: No, worsens it.

Danny Green, 46: On-the-job exercise does.

Brunhilda, 44: I go through stages—walking, weight lifting, and other forms of exercise. For right now, I'm trying step aerobics, but the choreography is so difficult, I procrastinate.

Zelda, 48: Since I am diabetic they have "put a gun" to my head. In other words, choose between feet and eyes, and the sofa.

Will, 38: I'm a lazy slob. At 295 pounds, I looked the role. At 245 – 260, I pass for hefty, but strong and more fit.

Jane, 53: I do think that exercise can help one recover from mental illness. I do not always exercise, but when I do, I like to walk, swim, or lift weights.

> Regular aerobic exercise improves mood and sleep, reduces stress and anxiety and raises self-esteem (Miller 49). Increasing oxygen to the brain also provides "better nourished" brain cells improving cognition (Carmichael 38).

Barnaby, 23: Exercise works wonders. I love to ride my bicycle, and the more I do, the better I feel. Before riding, my head will be cluttered; I might be depressed or stressed. Afterward, my head is clear and thinking becomes easier. My body feels good too. I highly recommend anyone with any mental illness to do some sort of exercise.

Harriet, 43: It is critical, but I don't exercise much. I do walk.

Ozzie, 46: I do a lot of walking, pushing carts at Harris Teeter.

Jill, 27: It makes me feel better about myself as well as controls the weight issue. I walk and swim.

Aileen, 54: Exercise helps you feel better. I walk most days.

Black Madonna, 36: I walk for a mile in place, or I may go walking around the block in my

Aerobic exercise prompts the release of mood lifting hormones and neurotransmitters like serotonin, which helps give people a sense of wellbeing and reduces stress (Miller 49, 55).

neighborhood.

Christen, 44: I suffer from leg pain; it hurts so bad sometimes that I can't walk. I started walking for exercise when I can, because the doctors won't give me pain medicine. It is helping. The pain is not as bad when I pray.

Brian, 43: Exercise is very helpful in my recovery because it helps me to feel better physically which helps me feel better emotionally. I mainly like to walk a lot and low-impact cardiovascular exercise.

Jay, 56: It helps a lot. Walking.

Rachel, 44: I exercise for recreation, health, weight control, and socialization.

Liana, 50: I like to swim—I think it is an aerobic way to experience thinking. I also like to walk.

Do you eat nutritiously? Why or why not?

Jade, 43: Yes, because it is important to my general health.

Socrates, 43: Since I work part time, I have enough money to eat nutritiously.

Adam, 28: Sort of.

Danny Green, 46: I do now.

Brunhilda, 44: I am currently on the South Beach diet with my boyfriend. It is the ultimate diet for people with schizophrenia. (We are scientifically categorized as "apples" and "carbohydrate addicts." This diet targets the stomach area and lowers carbohydrate intake.) I've lost 24 pounds on the South Beach diet. Before the diet I lost a half-pound/week without even trying, due to a reduction in medication. I don't consider stage one of the South Beach diet nutritious, but we're on stage three and eating more nutritiously than ever.

Zelda, 48: Yes, through my mother.

Will, 38: Hey, I'm the working poor. Besides, who has time to eat. Well, I must confess, I manage to both find the time and the money to keep myself well nourished.

Jane, 53: I think that I eat fairly nutritiously. My mother plans nutritious dinners, and this helps a lot. I also take some care about what I eat for the rest of the day. It does not seem too hard to eat nutritiously.

Barnaby, 23: I do eat lots of good foods; I just eat the bad ones too. Sometimes, if I'm in a bad mood, I'll use that as an excuse to eat whatever I want—sometimes chocolate helps.

Harriet, 43: Yes, but I am trying to eat better.

Ozzie, 46: Sometimes yes and no. I take a lot of vitamins and minerals.

Larry, 46: No, it is hard to cook at work and then cook at home at night.

Jill, 27: I try, but I don't like certain foods.

Aileen, 54: Yes, my housemate insists.

Black Madonna, 36: Yes! I try to eat plenty of fruits and vegetables. A lot. I have tried to cut back on chocolate and soda.

> Taking antipsychotics causes a person to lose the feeling of fullness they used to get at the end of an ordinary meal. This is one reason why people with schizophrenia tend to gain weight on these medications (Duckworth 4).

Christen, 44: Yes, because I am a diabetic, and so is my husband.

Brian, 43: I do eat nutritiously to an extent. I find that my limited financial budget makes it hard to afford healthy foods.

Jay, 56: Yes, for my health.

Rachel, 44: I try to be vegetarian when buying groceries, but because I need to rely on food pantries, I can't be too selective. My diabetes doctor suggested that I tell the food pantries that I am diabetic. I've tried it once, and it seems to have helped.

Liana, 50: Probably not. I drink too much Diet Coke, and I'm hooked on Wendy's Frosties.

Have you had any problems with substance abuse or dependence?

Jade, 43: As a child, but not as an adult.

Socrates, 43: Before my illness, I abused both alcohol and marijuana.

Adam, 28: Yes, drinking, pot.

Will, 38: Some experimentation nearly 20 years ago. Could have precipitated a decline.

> Use of street drugs (such as methamphetamine, LSD, and especially marijuana) has been linked with significantly increased risk of developing schizophrenia. One expert suggests that adding drug use to a previous disposition increases one's risk tenfold (www.schizophrenia.com).

Barnaby, 23: In high school I would drink and smoke marijuana and abuse the Adderall prescribed to me. I haven't done either of those drugs in years though (marijuana or Adderall). More recently, I used to abuse Oxycontin. It's a good thing I can't get that any more. I know it's not really a good thing to use opiates, but it's the best escape I know. That's really what drugs were about with me, an escape. I still drink occasionally, but alcohol doesn't help the intermittent cravings I get for something stronger. Drugs like that really change you, and I don't think you can go back.

Ozzie, 46: Yes, I used to drink a lot of beer.

Jill, 27: Yes, but I've been clean for five-and-a-half-months.

Black Madonna, 36: Yes! I have in the past. I have tried marijuana.

Liana, 50: I tried cocaine five times in 1985 but I act as is.

Which substances do you use, and how frequently do you use them?

Jade, 43: Caffeine—four cups a day.

Socrates, 43: I now smoke a couple of cigars a day and drink alcohol in moderation, perhaps once or twice a week. I also enjoy coffee.

Adam, 28: Cigarettes, a pack a day. Coffee twice a week. Alcohol twice a week.

Danny Green, 46: Two cups of coffee a day; four beers a week.

Brunhilda, 44: Nicotine—two packs a day. Coffee—one to two pots a day. Alcohol, diet pills, and street drugs make my illness worse. I drink two or three beers or wine coolers a year, so I don't feel like I'm missing anything.

Zelda, 48: Tea (caffeine) and cigarettes once a week.

Will, 38: Lots of java. Where would a large, hairy, muscular 250-pound man be without the occasional beer?

Jane, 53: I rarely have a caffeine drink. I used to have it much more often than I do now.

Barnaby, 23: I am a pretty heavy smoker and coffee drinker. I drink alcohol sometimes but usually not enough to get drunk.

> Approximately 85% of people who have schizophrenia are also heavy smokers, and they smoke two to three times as much as the average smoker. It is estimated that 44% of cigarettes smoked in the U.S. are smoked by people with mental illness (www.schizophrenia.com).

Harriet, 43: Caffeine in the morning. Alcohol rarely now, but I did drink in the past.

Ozzie, 46: I just drink coffee in the morning.

Jill, 27: Nicotine every five minutes; caffeine daily; alcohol, morphine and marijuana, but not any more.

Aileen, 54: Caffeine—two to four cups a day. Alcohol—one to two cups of wine, one to three times a week.

Black Madonna, 36: I do not use any substances at this time—I stopped months ago.

Christen, 44: I drink a lot of soda—nothing else.

Brian, 43: I do not currently smoke but did so for 20 years and have quit now for 12 years. I drink coffee and tea, and I no longer drink or use drugs but did to a great extent in the past.

Rachel, 44: Caffeine—three cups of regular coffee in the morning.

Liana, 50: I use caffeine in Diet Coke. I drink about five a day. I get codeine from someone concentrating 24 hours a day.

How have substances appeared to impact your illness?

Jade, 43: They keep me alert.

Socrates, 43: I believe caffeine helps me wake up and focus better. Nicotine also stimulates me and yet relaxes me as well. Alcohol often reduces anxiety and helps me relax also.

Brunhilda, 44: I like smoking and coffee because they're "as needed" and under my control. They control my mood level as well as clarity of mind.

Zelda, 48: Smoking helps the day go on.

Will, 38: Coffee in the a.m., beer with friends on occasion to unwind. Rarely do I drink when alone or in a bad mood/angry.

Jane, 53: When I was on another medicine than my present one, Zyprexa, my psychiatrist recommended caffeine to keep me from sleeping altogether too much. Other than that, I have had complete freedom to abstain from substances as I wished.

Barnaby, 23: Some drugs don't seem to impact my illness—alcohol for example. Other drugs, marijuana and Adderall, exacerbate my symptoms. Cigarettes, whether because of the direct action of nicotine or because they're calming for some other reason, help. I don't think I'll smoke marijuana again. I remember I was smoking with a friend; with the first puff it was like the voices were turned on. It was like flipping a light switch. Scary.

Harriet, 43: Hangovers are worse on meds.

Ozzie, 46: I think the beer I used to drink assisted in my mental illness.

Larry, 46: My usage was life-threatening for years until I found AA, NA. Even then it was about 12 years of off-and-on usage that continued to threaten me. I now have about 11 years of substance-free life.

Jill, 27: They used to make me crazier, so I had to quit. Except, of course, nicotine and caffeine.

Aileen, 54: They don't.

Black Madonna, 36: It made me paranoid.

> Many people with schizophrenia smoke, and it appears they get the same effects as others who report enjoying cigarettes: reduced anxiety, sedation and improved concentration. In addition, people with schizophrenia also appear to experience an improvement in brain function (Torrey 274).

Christen, 44: A little soda never hurt anybody.

Brian, 43: I used substances to self-medicate and "drown my sorrows." And substance abuse made my depression much worse and even caused me to become suicidal, leading to frequent hospitalizations.

Rachel, 44: Caffeine takes away some of the sleepiness.

Liana, 50: I'm hooked on codeine, and when I don't get it, I feel desperate about my weight.

Elaborations...

Zelda, 48: My family knew the wife of a Turkish diplomat who was in Hospital St. Anne. We are not sure whether she drank or not. I do remember her drinking wine at our house during dinner. You see this is the problem. Wine is an agricultural product/food in France, and not a drug, so their definition of substance abuse is different than ours.

I spent five years of my life in Paris, and schizophrenia and substance abuse is the sort of thing that fascinates me.

Schizophrenics have the right to smoke cigarettes. I am not sure whether it is smart. There are some who contend that tobacco helps with the symptoms of the condition. Ask the tobacco smoker-schizophrenics around you.

Media and Interests

The greatness of an artist lies in the building of an inner world, and in the ability to reconcile the inner world with the outer.

– Albert Einstein

Sojourn in Winter

– Chris Yount

A melodic vigor penetrates this quiet mind
As adipose awareness feeds mealtime inspiration
In quest of comfort at the realization
That this sun-starved winter is a season too
A season made to wander

I stand outside the back door
Flicking icicles with my index finger
A single-shot vibraphone hanging from the rain gutter
Rusting just above my head

The pitches of these fangs in winter
Pierce through me as I march uphill
Into fields and forests
Guarding their myriad secrets until they succumb
To the gossip of springtime thaw

But all these secrets do drip
They drip outside my own back door
Revealed to me every morning before coffee
As I repeat the pitches made known
By the clear white fangs of winter.

What is your favorite factual book on mental illness? Your favorite fiction book? Your favorite movie?

Jade, 43: *Touched with Fire*, by Kay Redfield Jamison; *The Butcher Boy*; *Benny & Joon*.

Socrates, 43: My favorite book on mental illness is Mark Vonnegut's *Eden Express*. My favorite fiction book on mental illness is Ken Kesey's *One Flew Over the Cuckoo's Nest*. And my favorite movie is *A Beautiful Mind*.

Adam, 28: Fiction: *Heart of Darkness* and *Crime and Punishment*. Movie: *Apocalypse Now*.

Danny Green, 46: Factual: *Darkness Visible*, Styron; Fiction: *One Flew Over the Cuckoo's Nest*, Kesey and *Ward 6*, Checkov; Movie: *Harvey*.

Brunhilda, 44: Factual – *Surviving Schizophrenia* by E. Fuller Torrey. Personal experience novel (not fiction) – *The Quiet Room* by Lori Schiller and Amanda Bennett. Movie (fictional) – *Caveman's Valentine*.

Zelda, 48: Books: E Fuller Torrey's *Surviving Schizophrenia*. Movies: *One Flew Over the Cuckoo's Nest* and *A Beautiful Mind*.

Will, 38: Nonfiction: What else, the DSM-IV-TR! *The Bible*, stories fact or fiction. Movies: *One Flew Over the Cuckoo's Nest* and *Girl, Interrupted*.

Jane, 53: I do not have a favorite factual book about mental illness or a favorite novel. I did see and mostly like the movie *March of the Penguins* when it was showing.

Barnaby, 23: I don't know many factual books on mental illness, just the DSM. My favorite fiction book is Albert Camus' *The Plague*. Before I got sick, before I believed in God, I was a big fan of the French existentialists. The idea that there isn't anything more to the universe beyond the simple fact that it exists was both depressing and appealing, empowering really. Now I think the opposite: believing in God and the spiritual is the only answer to an inscrutable world.

Harriet, 43: No favorite book. My favorite movie is *A Beautiful Mind*.

Ozzie, 46: I don't have any favorite book. I watch a lot of movies, and I like westerns.

Larry, 46: *Eden Express. Girl, Interrupted.*

Jill, 27: *Eden Express, Catch 22,* and *Rain Man.*

Aileen, 54: My favorite fictional book is *The White Dragon* by Anne McCaffrey. My favorite movie is *Sirens*.

Black Madonna, 36: *The Day the Voices Stopped.* I do not have a favorite movie or a favorite fiction book.

Christen, 44: I don't read many books because of my illness. I like *A Beautiful Mind* as a movie.

Brian, 43: My favorite book on mental illness is *Surviving Schizophrenia* by E. Fuller Torrey. My favorite fiction book is *Dune*, and my favorite movie is *A Beautiful Mind*.

Jay, 56: *Zen and the Art of Motocycle Maintenance. A Beautiful Mind.*

Rachel, 44: My favorite book on mental illness is *I Know This Much is True* by Wally Lamb.

Liana, 50: My favorite book is *Eden Express*. Favorite movie is *The Three Faces of Eve.*

How does your mental illness affect you when you travel?

Jade, 43: I get stressed on plane trips.

Socrates, 43: I find I don't like to spend too long away from home where I can be in my natural rhythm of things. I enjoy visiting family, but more than a week away is too much.

Danny Green, 46: All who dream and desire to travel should follow their dreams. One should minimize stress and be sure one has enough food, medicine, and lodging.

Brunhilda, 44: I travel as little as possible. It just seems the farther I travel, the more likely I hallucinate or become ill. Because I'm on Medicaid, I feel insecure about whether I can receive treatment out of state or country.

Zelda, 48: Constant juggle with meds.

Will, 38: I think travel is stressful for anyone, even people who do it for a living.

A 1989 study found that 68% of outpatients with schizophrenia drive versus 99% of the control group without mental disorders. Drivers with schizophrenia are usually adept at "operational coordination," yet some are impaired in "planning," "tactical decisions," "judgment" and "paying attention" (Torrey 361-2).

Jane, 53: I don't want to fly. I don't want to drive on I-40 where the traffic can be terrible. Sometimes I've had to drive on 15-501 to church gatherings. That seems to take a special kind of courage. When my parents and I are going somewhere, one of them usually drives, and I spend the time in much silent prayer. I do not like that many drivers speed and do not signal when they intend to change lanes! I pray to be a safe driver, and that prayer has been graciously answered; I have no violations on my record.

Barnaby, 23: My symptoms get worse when I travel, especially in airports. There is so little stimulus and so little to do in airports that sometimes all I could do was listen to the voices. It can get that way in planes, too. Aside from that, being in hotels is kind of depressing.

Harriet, 43: Anxious leaving my parents. I can handle it well with meds.

Larry, 46: I need to pay attention to spending less time alone than I do at home.

Jill, 27: It depends on if I'm having symptoms. There is always anxiety.

Aileen, 54: I am a little more nervous, especially before I get there. I have to rest more than other people.

Black Madonna, 36: I do not take long trips because I feel anxiety.

Christen, 44: Being in a plane or car stresses me out too much.

Brian, 43: I have a great deal of anxiety when I am in airports. I am very nervous while checking in and going through security.

Rachel, 44: Being with a different set of people and a different schedule is difficult, but I love seeing family.

Liana, 50: I like being in motion.

What are your interests or hobbies, and how much time do you spend on them?

Jade, 43: Music an hour a day; poetry an hour a day; swimming an hour a day.

Socrates, 43: I enjoy reading (two hours/day), writing (two-to-three hours weekly), exercising (one hour/day), and an occasional golf outing.

Adam, 28: Watching sports, three-to-six hours a day; video games four hours a day; reading two hours a day.

Danny Green, 46: Natural history; political science; writing; chess; gardening; hiking; literature; music; faith. Now, all of my time.

Brunhilda, 44: My hobbies are drawing, painting, all types of crafts, and gardening in my relatives' yards, as well as having a vegetable garden. The time I spend on them varies greatly due to the project. I have a disorder of attention so I don't read much.

Zelda, 48: I sleep and paint.

Will, 38: Writing and music. Not enough.

Jane, 53: I spend half an hour, or a little more, reading the Bible daily. Sometimes I go walking and observing

> While it may be that people with mental illness are more creative than the general population, it is often associated with the high productivity of a manic episode in bipolar disorder. In 1980, a review of past studies indicated that people with schizophrenia are no more likely to be creative than the general population (Noll 111).

the birds; in our neighborhood, there are often songbirds. My parents like to have the television on when there is something in which one of their grandchildren is interested. The current "thing" is ice hockey. I don't particularly like it. It seems too much like a brawl sometimes, but I try to be a good sport about it, since my parents are interested.

Barnaby, 23: Most of my hobbies are such that I can escape into a different world, a fantasy world. When I get the chance, I role play; I play Magic; I play a tabletop strategy game called Warhammer. Aside from these rather nerdy-sounding games, I like paintball because it's so intense. I write a lot of poems too. I'd say these activities take up a good bit of time; more days than not I do something involving one of them.

Harriet, 43: Shopping, eating, socializing.

Ozzie, 46: I like to watch movies and listen to CDs. I spend approximately two-to-four hours a week.

Jill, 27: Writing short stories and poetry. I also enjoy dabbling with web design. It depends on how I'm feeling. On average, two hours a day.

Aileen, 54: Ceramics—two-to-four hours/week. Painting—three-to-five hours/month. Reading—daily. Crochet—most days. Sudoku—daily. Other puzzles—two-to-three times/week. Croquet—one-to-two times each summer.

Black Madonna, 36: Writing in my journal, reading, self-help books—school on-line—I am studying business.

Christen, 44: My favorite things to do are shopping, listening to gospel music, going to church and talking on the phone.

Brian, 43: I watch a lot of movies and spend several hours a week watching movies. I also like to read and spend time on my computer on the internet.

Jay, 56: Reading—several hours a day.

Liana, 50: I used to play the flute and was told I had potential, but I stopped playing and now I can't read music any more. I also like ping pong, and like to water ski. For an indefinite amount of time.

Does your illness encourage or restrict you from certain types of media? Which types of media do you prefer or avoid (if any)?

Jade, 43: I listen to the radio; I go on line; I read the *New Yorker*, *Granta*, *Rolling Stone*, and *Poetry*; I watch some TV (cooking shows and *Law and Order*).

Socrates, 43: Not really. Sometimes commercials (both radio and TV) grate on my nerves.

Adam, 28: I avoid TV comedy and night-time radio.

> Lack of concentration is both a symptom of the illness and a side-effect of medications, and it affects people's ability to enjoy leisure activities such as reading and watching (Miller and Mason 68).

Brunhilda, 44: In my original mental illness I listened to the radio 24/7 so I wouldn't feel alone. Now I can't stand radio, especially rude morning shows. Now I watch movies, read the papers. I don't like TV news or certain TV shows, and still I feel I watch too much violence.

Zelda, 48: I am a news-aholic so I listen to NPR and CNN.

Will, 38: As far as I am concerned, advocacy by consumers is a way of life. I don't watch much TV.

Jane, 53: I don't like war movies. I generally avoid fiction. I don't particularly like rock music. Too much of any kind of noise makes me unhappy. I don't like too many news shows. I almost never like commercials and often find them detestably boring.

Barnaby, 23: I don't avoid any type of media. I can tell you, though, that a few years ago I thought God was picking specific, meaningful songs to play for me on the radio. I would listen and try to figure out what he was telling me. You can pretty much hear what you want to hear when interpreting songs and trying to figure out how they reflect on you.

Harriet, 43: I enjoy radio, magazines, and movies. I avoid TV news.

Larry, 46: At one time, media was very difficult to incorporate into my life. Today I have difficulty with newspapers and magazines, due to concentration problems.

Jill, 27: Lots of times my illness restricts me from TV, especially when I have delusions. I prefer books and reading.

Aileen, 54: I prefer TV and movies. I avoid news, especially on TV.

Black Madonna, 36: TV when I'm manic—because I feel like I am communicating with the TV, or the TV is communicating with me.

Christen, 44: I read the Bible and listen to gospel music. I don't like TV, music, or books.

> Common delusional scenarios are being wired or radio controlled, thought broadcasting, being followed or watched, or that a famous person is in love with the individual. Media plays an important role in paranoid delusions and delusions of reference. For example, delusions centered around the internet have become more common (Torrey 28).

Brian, 43: My illness does not restrict me from media except that I do not like to read newspapers because they depress me. Otherwise I like to watch the news on TV such as CNN or MSNBC, etc. I hate movies.

Liana, 50: I prefer Weight Watchers' magazine to any of the other types of media. I like popular music. I avoid TV news. I have a favorite movie I saw in 1974—they showed it on television in 1977, but they won't show it again.

Elaborations...

Aileen, 54: Because of the "Brushes with Life" artist program with UNC Hospitals, I have had more opportunities to show my work than I would have otherwise.

Brunhilda, 44: Most of my friends with schizophrenia travel a lot. They always ask me why I don't travel more. There appears to be a direct correlation between the further I travel and also the duration of the trip with the greater chance and the severity of becoming ill.

Many years ago, in college I had my money lifted while I was in Paris. I spent days on end wandering around aimlessly through the ugly "blue-light district," listening to my constant companions, "the voices." I had no money for the metro or cigarettes.

Gradually, I had become significantly ill over a long period of time, probably due to multiple overdosing attempts. It all culminated later in England when I lay in bed for five straight days. The whole time I only got up for infrequent smoking until I ran out, to drink water and to go to the bathroom. All I did was listen to the voices shout at me. You know you have it bad when the voices won't stop screaming!

More recently, there was an incident on my return flight from a family reunion in San Diego. The night before we were leaving to return, I got in an argument with my mother. The whole time at the airports and on the planes I would see and hear the actual comments strangers would say to each other, yet their voices, repeatedly, sounded like members of my family. I attempted to ground myself in reality, when I realized at the baggage claim, it wasn't possible to hear my sister's voice 25 feet away, because I couldn't make out what the guy standing next to me was saying.

Last year, on the first night of our annual camping trip, I awoke at 3 a.m. and urgently stumbled to the bathroom. It was very dark, and I have no sense of direction anyway. I proceeded in getting very lost. For a long time, I wandered around tripping on all the speed bumps. Just as the sun was rising, I came out of my medicated stupor, and suddenly I was clear headed, and not only did I know the names of all the roads, I instantaneously recalled the exact campsite numbers. What happened? I still don't know.

The System & Financial Concerns

Poverty is the open-mouthed relentless hell which yawns beneath civilized society.

– Henry George

Riding the Bipolar Roller Coaster

– Colette Corr

Climbing out of the depth of dark despair
Watching the sunrise with reinvigorated hope
Cycling upward and upward
Within hours completing
The bipolar roller coaster ride

Over and over, up and down
Beginning with depressive nothingness
Leading to the creative rush
Following with few productive hours
Bursting into mania
Impairing concentration and ability to sit still
Crashing exhausted into long, deep sleep
Reluctantly, waking up
Coffee, the only readily available solution

Are you on disability? How old were you when you qualified? How many years had you been ill before going on disability?

Jade, 43: Yes—34. I'm not sure.

Socrates, 43: I receive SSDI. I suffered for eight years before I ever knew about SSDI. I have received assistance since I was 36 years old.

Adam, 28: Yes, 25 years old, three years.

Danny Green, 46: Yes, 38. Twenty-one years.

Brunhilda, 44: I qualified for disability at 32 years old. I had been ill for 12 years previously. I had tried and failed at so many jobs it was easy to get disability. When I qualified, it was based on my preceding restaurant wage of $2.15/hour.

Zelda, 48: Yes, 43, I think.

Will, 38: No (although I was before). Thirty years. Fifteen years.

Jane, 53: I am on SSI. When I qualified, I was in my 40s. I had been ill for some years before I was on SSI.

Barnaby, 23: I am on disability and have been for two years. I think I was 21 when I qualified. I'd been ill three years before I applied. There was definitely a time when I couldn't have worked. Now I think I could if I had to. I'm thinking maybe I don't need it any more.

Harriet, 43: Yes, since 1996. I was 33 and had been sick for 15 years.

Ozzie, 46: Yes. I was 38. I was ill three years before disability.

Larry, 46: No.

Jill, 27: Yes. 18. 15.

Aileen, 54: Yes. 52. Ten years.

Black Madonna, 36: Yes, since I was 27. Twelve years.

Christen, 44: I was 25 when I first became ill. When I first went on disability I can't remember—it's been such a long time.

> **Social Security Disability Insurance** (SSDI) is provided by the U.S. government. To be eligible for benefits, a person must be unable to work, due to disability, for 12 months.
> **Supplemental Security Income** (SSI) is for people who were not working when they became disabled. A need-based benefit, SSI is intended for people with no significant work history and few financial resources.

Brian, 43: Yes, I receive SSI and SSDI. I was 27 years old when I qualified, and I had been sick for six years before getting it.

Jay, 56: Yes. Thirty years old. Four years.

Liana, 50: Yes, I'm on disability—I was 25 when I was qualified. I wasn't even ill.

How has the need for high-priced medications changed your life, if at all?

Jade, 43: It is blowing my security to pieces—this Medicare system.

Socrates, 43: The cost of my medication is in excess of $800/month. Every year I worry I will lose my disability and not be able to afford my meds. Before I got SSDI, I paid for my meds (I worked two jobs despite severe illness at the time), but they were cheaper then ($250/month). I used to feel I was in a financial box that was impossible to break out of. I no longer feel that way because my life goals have changed. I am more focused on internals rather than externals.

Adam, 28: Hasn't yet because of health plan coverage.

Danny Green, 46: It's eaten into earnings and savings.

Brunhilda, 44: Disability and Medicaid totally changed my life. Without it, I wouldn't have received my high-priced medications and would have kept failing at full-time jobs I wasn't capable of.

Zelda, 48: I need to maintain my benefits.

Will, 38: My brain is a wild animal, and I kind of like it that way. Meds help but not without some hindrances as well.

Jane, 53: I want to be careful what kind of job I get, so that either I can keep Medicaid or I will be able to purchase my medicine on my own. Actually, I have felt somewhat flattered to be on state-of-the-art medicine, when this has been so.

> People who receive SSDI become eligible for Medicare benefits, including the prescription drug plans, after 24 months (Miller and Mason 156).

Barnaby, 23: With my insurance, the medications are actually pretty cheap. Taking medications in general is a nightly reminder of how sick I've been and am.

Harriet, 43: Medicare and Medicaid are most helpful.

Ozzie, 46: I changed to a generic prescription based on the doctor's advice.

Jill, 27: I have to watch my budget. Thank God for my parents.

Aileen, 54: So far there has been no effect but I'm afraid that will change when I qualify for Medicare. *(Many medication assistance programs are not available to people who have prescription coverage.)*

Black Madonna, 36: High-priced medications have drained me financially, but I receive Medicare and Humana now. This has helped me tremendously.

Christen, 44: My life has changed a lot because of the need to get my medicine. We wouldn't have been able to afford a car if someone hadn't given us one. We have a very strict budget with very few extras.

Brian, 43: To a great degree. I cannot afford to pay for my medication and therefore must stay on my benefits to pay for them. If I did not need assistance to pay for them, or if I had a good insurance policy, I could then work full time.

Rachel, 44: They're almost completely paid for by Medicaid.

Liana, 50: I've never experienced drugs as being extravagant.

What are your financial restrictions?

Jade, 43: I live on a very fixed income.

Socrates, 43: I work part time and receive SSDI and Medicare. I live very frugally, but I am more fortunate than most people with my illness because I have employment.

Danny Green, 46: It seems I can no longer work full time.

Brunhilda, 44: My finances are manageable, but I need a part-time job for extras in life. Having a little more spending money makes life more bearable.

Zelda, 48: I am too broke to move. I can't get a credit card.

Will, 38: Everybody has a budget, even the President of the US, and he's more in debt than I am, yes?

Jane, 53: I cannot have $2000 or more.

Barnaby, 23: Living with my parents, I thankfully don't have to worry about that too much. I can't go on a shopping spree, but I have everything I need.

Harriet, 43: I am poor.

Ozzie, 46: Medicare now covers my medicine, and I pay a $5 co-pay.

Larry, 46: Being employed for the last 10 years has opened up a world of possibilities for me financially.

Jill, 27: I have been blessed—I have everything that I need.

Aileen, 54: I can't make too much money. There's a limit for disability and the financial aid program with the hospital. Financial restrictions are very important. I've had to limit my income to qualify for programs that can help me with my finances. This has made some difficulties for me.

Black Madonna, 36: I can't buy a car now, or move into a new home, until after bankruptcy.

Brian, 43: I live off of a very small amount of money each month, and even though I work part time I can barely afford to pay for gas for my car and keep in a good supply of groceries. It is very hard to make ends meet on my limited budget.

Jay, 56: Not much spending money.

Rachel, 44: I eat from food pantries. I have very little money for entertainment or food. I don't spend money on clothes, and I usually can choose one thing from about six new needs that come up each month.

Liana, 50: I can only buy clothes when they're half off at the thrift store. I can't afford Weight Watchers.

Are you concerned about the stability of Social Security benefits? Why or why not?

Jade, 43: Definitely. A lot of people rely on those benefits.

Socrates, 43: I think we should be very concerned about future benefits. Our national debt is out of control, and with baby boomers soon to retire, the strain on our budget may result in cuts to Social Security, Medicaid and Medicare.

Danny Green, 46: Since Domenici-Kennedy Americans with Disabilities Act, I hope not.

Will, 38: Unfortunately, yes. I lost my SSI and Medicaid slightly before I should have. Uncle Sam cut me off in graduate school. The guy should have waited for me to work and pay taxes until I proved myself to me, not to him.

Jane, 53: I think the Good Lord has done a very good job of keeping me from getting really anxious about all the national debt and deficit! I do feel concerned when I hear about "baby-boomers" who are in their late 60s and still have to work to maintain their lifestyles. As they get older, people can get more vulnerable to health problems. I am also concerned for all the previous children who are getting born and growing up, because of the problems with which I hope the Lord defends them from getting stuck! Nevertheless, I am sure that the Lord Jesus can take care of my concerns.

Harriet, 43: Yes, who isn't? I hate Bush.

Ozzie, 46: Yes, I'm afraid of being cut off. They evaluate me every three years. If I make too much money part time, they can cut me off.

Larry, 46: Yes, if I ever have to go back on Social Security, I would want it to be available.

Jill, 27: Yes, because North Carolina is making some changes.

Aileen, 54: Yes, I'm concerned because I'm dependent on them.

Black Madonna, 36: Yes! There may not be enough money left for seniors in years to come.

Christen, 44: I hope they'll always be there. If not, a lot of people are in trouble.

Brian, 43: Yes, I am concerned because the rules regarding holding a job while on benefits are so strict that you would lose your benefits if you work too much.

Jay, 56: Yes, I need my monthly check to survive.

Liana, 50: Yes—they must know that I won't work because I'm fat.

What changes would like to see made in the services for the mentally ill?

Jade, 43: An income for the mentally ill and guaranteed, state-sponsored medication.

Socrates, 43: I think the system is grossly unfair to most of the mentally ill. Many of my friends are expected to live on $500 or $600 a month. Though some of them have reduced rent, it is still very difficult to live on such a low budget. I think that the minimum benefit should be increased, and the maximum amount someone can earn raised. Just because you have a mental illness, should you be delegated to poverty?

Adam, 28: More parity in benefits.

Danny Green, 46: Poverty and mental illness seem inextricably bound together, whether fair or unfair. We just need our medicine, food, and housing.

Brunhilda, 44: 1. Disability applications and reviews specifically written for the mentally ill. 2. Acknowledgements that reviewing work history from 10 years ago has nothing to do with current situations and mental competency. 3. A new system recalculating how much disability entitlement should be given, by recalculating the date the person became ill, not by the date of the application.

Zelda, 48: Tons—we need national health insurance.

Will, 38: Parity, secure community-based services. If our budget for mental health resembled the money going to Iraq, we'd be in great shape. Put a minority female in office who is good friends with Rosalyn Carter and Tipper Gore.

Jane, 53: I would like to be able to have more money in savings than I now have. I once had a very hard time getting some dental work done, and I currently have a situation with my car, which I do not know how much it will take to repair. I would like to have a medicine which would make it very much easier to lose weight and to keep it off. I would like to be treated more as though other people knew that the Lord could heal me, and not as though I necessarily had some kind of lifetime problem. I have been feeling better lately, and I do not know all the reasons why. I have been on my medicine for a few years now, so I do not think it is the medicine.

Barnaby, 23: I'd like to see hospital inpatient programs improved to the point where they don't feel like prisons. I admit I don't know how to do that, but surely something could change. Being in a psych ward can actually make my symptoms worse, which is woefully counterproductive.

Harriet, 43: More stability in the system.

Ozzie, 46: I would like to see a guaranteed disability and Medicare. Since it is a fearful situation being cut off of social security.

Larry, 46: More focus on housing and access for the new medications to be available for all who need them.

Jill, 27: Better hospitals, better insurance.

Aileen, 54: Low-cost, high-quality meds.

Black Madonna, 36: More jobs; education; help the homeless community; advocacy. And those who are in jail who have mental illness, also those who abuse drugs and alcohol who have a mental illness; more education, classes. I would like to see more people who have mental illness in Congress and the legislative community, and the Senate, passing more laws for the cause of advocacy for those with disabilities. I would like to see more club houses. I would like to see the homeless who are mentally ill get help. Those who abuse drugs and alcohol get help if they are mentally ill. Those who are incarcerated or in jail get the help they need; they are often thrown in jail without being screened for depression or mental illness. They never get the help they need. I am really concerned for those with mental illness who are homeless and behind bars. Those on drugs and alcohol who often use drugs to cover up their mental illness.

Christen, 44: Bigger check, of course.

Brian, 43: I would like to see a wider variety of services. Currently there are too few choices of services for people with mental illness. Currently you can choose between clubhouse or therapy, and that's all.

Jay, 56: More funds for rehab activities.

Rachel, 44: I would like to see a greater variety of housing options for the mentally ill in the area. I would like to see more discount programs for the disabled, especially in technology, which the poor cannot afford.

Liana, 50: More transactional analysis as therapy for depression.

Elaborations...

Socrates, 44: The financial picture for the mentally ill is not a pretty one. For the first nine years of my illness, I did not know about disability for someone in my circumstance, and it took 13 hospitalizations, homelessness, a good social worker and a non-profit organization to finally get it. Now that I have disability, I fear losing it because my condition has improved. Losing disability would mean losing Medicare, which would make it impossible for me to get my medication. This is the situation all of us with a preexisting illness face.

I had to try nearly a dozen medications to find one that actually worked and didn't give me awful side effects. Sometimes the side effects from some of these meds are as bad as the illness. If you've ever had akathisia you know what I'm talking about. It's like restless leg syndrome throughout your entire body. The medication that works for me is Zyprexa at the tune of $660 a month—that's $22 a pill. How many of us can throw away $22 a day on one pill? My other meds aren't cheap, but really, isn't this picture a little ridiculous?

And I am one of the fortunate ones. I have been able to hold the same part-time job for nine years. Some of my fellow sufferers can't even find work. You try finding a job with a checkered work history that mental illness inevitably creates. Or try being honest and telling a prospective employer about your illness. Though it's illegal to discriminate on the basis of one's illness, any employer will find another reason (though fictitious) not to hire you.

And my friends look down on me for being on the government docket. Try paying $900 a month on medication and supporting yourself on $20,000 a year. After taxes you may have $16,000 or $17,000 to live on. Subtract over $10,000 for meds, and you're down to $6,000, and that's without doctor bills. Have you ever tried to live on $6,000 a year? That's $500 a month. Even the worst-off of my friends with mental illness have more than that, and their rent is subsidized, and their treatment is free. Sound like a catch-22? You bet it is.

So, what am I going to do? I am going to risk losing everything and go back to school so I can get a job that is not too stressful, but will pay me enough and provide benefits, so I can afford my own meds. But most people with schizophrenia don't have this option. They either don't have the educational background or don't function at a high enough level to pull it off. The best they can hope for is a part-time job which will provide them enough money for tobacco and something other than oodles of noodles. And people begrudge them their disability. After you've walked a day in one of our shoes, then let's see what you have to say.

Danny Green, 46: Before I ever qualified for disability assistance, I struggled mightily to both earn my living and afford my medicine. When certain MDs and families refused to acknowledge my disability, things got progressively worse. My schooling ended prematurely with the onset of my diagnosis. So I was left with little training and scant opportunity. Although I remain ready and willing, the jobs I filled in my teens, 20s, 30s, and 40s involved work that current assertions insist "no American would do."

I spent the 21 years between being diagnosed at age 17 and my qualifying for disability assistance at age 38 doing everything in my power to keep my life afloat. There seems a powerful resistance on the part of society and many families to the fact that schizophrenia and schizoaffective disorder are pervasive, chronic and (generally) life-long conditions.

Money is the main reason most of us work. To house, clothe, and feed ourselves provide decisive and urgent incentives for us to remain in some form of gainful employment.

If you work full-time, you may well be unable to afford required medicine on your job's health plan. If you have no reliable health plan, you cannot get medicine. Without required medicine, you cannot work. This is the bind many of us face throughout our working lives. If we forsake the pride of earning our livings, we lose self-esteem, the esteem of our families, and that of society at large. So the stigma of joblessness compounds the stigma of mental illness. All that we can do is try to become as healthy as possible and remain in the game. And this includes finances.

To navigate the arcane twists and turns of SSI, SSDI, Medicaid, and Medicare, we must usually enlist the help of professionals. Personally, I am living on a yearly disability budget of $6,924. Because of this aid, I'm also able to afford a roughly equal dollar amount of medicine and therapy per annum. I never had this access to medical services when I worked full time. During those years I paid for my medicine out of pocket.

Stigma

It is no measure of health to be well adjusted to a profoundly sick society.

– Jiddu Krishnamurti

Ugliness and Society

– Danny Green

How ugly could it be that healthy
people can think up no
harsher put-down against other
healthy people than castigating
them with my diagnosis?

And murderers would use my
diagnosis to excuse themselves
from responsibility for their crimes,
when we who actually suffer
these diagnoses take full responsibility
for our disabilities.

What misconceptions do you think that people have about mental illness? Do people treat you differently when they learn about your illness?

Jade, 43: I think people think I'm a little strange, but I don't usually tell them I'm schizo. I just don't worry about it. They might have the same problem themselves.

Socrates, 43: I once told a woman in a bar that I suffered from schizoaffective disorder, and she asked me if I had multiple personalities. Up until I told her about my illness she seemed very interested in me. After I told her about my illness, she quickly left the bar.

Adam, 28: Ignorance about the entirety of my diagnosis. No.

> In the 18th Century, the first psychiatric hospital, which opened in 1377, allowed the public to watch the patients, who were billed as a "freak show," for a penny (Lunatic 6).

Brunhilda, 44: One time my mother knew I was delusional and probably hallucinating and made me stay in bed. My sister brought me breakfast in bed. How ridiculous! Most people, when they find out, act like you have cooties!

Zelda, 48: That if one is a schizophrenic with a profession, they tend to patronize you when they find out you can speak professionally.

Jane, 53: I think that people are often afraid of insanity in another person. I don't know if people treat me differently when they know about my mental illness; I've often had difficulty making friends anyway.

Barnaby, 23: I've been written off before as "crazy." Some people seem to think that if you have a mental illness, you are not as worthwhile or not as much of a person as people without an illness. They dehumanize you with your diagnosis. As far as people learning about my illness,

181

the people who care are kind even if they don't understand. I had one friend who is scared of me now. I think that people with mental illnesses need to stay social with people they can trust. I lost a lot of social skills when I got sick, and the only way to get them back is to be with people.

Harriet, 43: I can't live a quality life—and it is hindered—I have some new friends that I haven't told.

Ozzie, 46: I think they have a hard time accepting it and say to themselves, "That would never happen to me." No, they don't treat me differently.

Larry, 46: I think a large percentage of the stigma can be an individual and internalized process that people with mental illness can bring on themselves. If you can't live with your illness, how can you experience others living with you?

Jill, 27: A lot of people think we are monsters or we are stupid. Some treat me differently, some do not.

Aileen, 54: They think they might get hurt. I'm careful who I tell, and I haven't been treated differently.

Black Madonna, 36: Yes – I feel like the church needs to get more involved with the mental health reform and the recovery for people who have mental illness. There is a big stigma in the church through my experience.

Christen, 44: I think most people think people with mental illness hurt people. I believe if they knew some of us, they would think differently.

Brian, 43: I think that most people think that people with mental illness are dangerous, which in the vast majority of cases is simply false.

I think that people can sense that I am different at times and feel uncomfortable around me.

Jay, 56: That those with mental illness cannot work with their minds.

Rachel, 44: The misconception that I have the most difficulty with is that a person with mental illness is somehow someone to pity that cannot be helpful to them. Often, before people find out about the illness, they blame other things that have nothing to do with the illness.

Liana, 50: The main misconception people have about mental illness is that mentally ill people are slow.

Whom have you told? What are your criteria that people must meet before you tell them you have a mental illness?

Jade, 43: My family knows. We're very tight.

Socrates, 43: I used to tell others, even strangers, about my illness, but I have learned that as soon as you tell them, their demeanor changes. Most people start to talk down to you when they find out you have a mental illness. They think you are unstable or inferior somehow. I no longer tell strangers that I have mental illness.

Adam, 28: My family. My friends. Complete trust and confidence.

Danny Green, 46: It never comes up—I'd tell everyone.

Brunhilda, 44: I don't tell many people. I just get paranoid that they can tell or heard it from someone else.

Will, 38: People I trust. People who watch TV. Whether someone knows or not, what they really need to pay attention to is how I have chosen to live my life.

Jane, 53: I have told almost no one that I have a mental illness, except for supervisors, when I have interviewed for jobs. One church friend knows. One prayer partner knows. Otherwise, I am not sure I have criteria for telling someone I have a mental illness. Thinking about it, I would tell a supervisor, and I would tell almost anyone who was what is called "born again" in Christian terms, if the person needed to know.

Barnaby, 23: I've told some friends and family; I've learned to be a little more close-mouthed about my illness. On the one hand, I'd like to tell certain people that I have schizoaffective disorder because it would help them understand me. On the other hand, no one would understand. I don't know what my criteria are, but I think they would have to broach the subject.

Harriet, 43: Outside the clubhouse, I have told a few neighbors. I am careful about this.

Ozzie, 46: They have to be trusting. My wife and her parents know. My brother and sister know.

> If a person with mental illness is deciding whether or not to tell someone about the diagnosis, some questions to ask might be: Will the person discover anyway? Does the person possess an educated understanding of schizophrenia? Will it change trust issues in the relationship (Torrey 365)?

Larry, 46: I normally don't tell others, but in some circumstances there is no way of getting around it.

Jill, 27: Most people that I get to know pretty well, I tell. My criterion is simply that I know the person.

Aileen, 54: On a need-to-know basis. My family, friends, employer, art teachers.

Black Madonna, 36: I have told the President of the U.S. about stigma and mental illness. They must have an open mind. I have told legislative persons – state and local.

Christen, 44: I don't need a reason to tell people. I just tell them because I am not ashamed of my illness.

Brian, 43: I do not hide the fact that I have a mental illness from anyone. I do not tell everyone, but if it comes up, I do not hide it, and I am not ashamed of it. I am completely "out of the closet" when it comes to my illness, and I do not stigmatize myself.

Jay, 56: People I encounter, when I want acceptance.

Rachel, 44: I tell my friends when I know they respect me as a friend.

Liana, 50: I got in an argument with a cashier in a grocery store in 1990 and got kicked out of the store and later told the manager it was because I didn't take my medication.

Is there anything that really gets on your nerves when people talk to you about mental illness?

Jade, 43: I don't like it when people say, "Are you getting hyper?"

Socrates, 43: Most people don't talk to me about my illness. If I didn't tell others, I don't think they would even know that I am mentally ill. I do a good job of hiding my symptoms.

Brunhilda, 44: I don't like it when they feel they have to talk to you as a child.

Zelda, 48: Being patronized.

Will, 38: Ignorant people are funny to me.

Jane, 53: When people call me crazy or speak as though I will always be this way, I can get irritated.

Barnaby, 23: It bugs me when people treat me like I'm not smart or when they walk on eggshells.

Harriet, 43: People who don't understand and are not educated about it.

Larry, 46: Bringing up too much of the past that there is nothing to be done about it, good or bad.

Jill, 27: When they tell me to use DBT skills when I am really mad.

Aileen, 54: I prefer it to be called a brain disorder.

Black Madonna, 36: When people use the word crazy a lot, loosely.

Christen, 44: It bothers me that some people who are mentally ill blame everything on their illness.

Brian, 43: It gets on my nerves only if the person who is talking to me knows nothing about it or if they have no idea what they are talking about. And I usually find that the people who know the most about it are the people who have experienced it.

Liana, 50: My sister-in-law said, "When you cough like that, it bothers me."

Which colloquial terms for mental illness do you dislike the most (for example, "loony tunes")?

Jade, 43: I don't dislike any of them. I take ownership of them. I rather like "loony tunes."

Socrates, 43: I kind of like "psycho," "off your rocker," and "head case."

Adam, 28: Mental case, basket case.

Danny Green, 46: I only object to people who use my diagnosis as a kind of pejorative against healthy people.

Brunhilda, 44: "La-la land." We're all having such a good time! Names related to fruit, including "fruit-loops."

Zelda, 48: Loony tunes, space cadet.

Will, 38: Sticks and stones...

In *Alice in Wonderland* written by Lewis Carroll in 1865, the character The Mad Hatter is believed to be based on professional hat makers of the period who used mercuric nitrate to block felt hats, which induced psychosis (Noll 275).

Jane, 53: You're right, I don't like "loony tunes!" I was called "a crazy person" once, and I didn't like that. Otherwise, I do not seem to have had any problems with being called bad names.

Barnaby, 23: I don't mind the terms—just when people use them in a demeaning way. The same statement can be insulting or statement of fact, depending on how it's said.

Harriet, 43: Crazy, sick, not well.

Ozzie, 46: Weirdo.

Larry, 46: At this point in time I don't pay much attention to labels, good or bad.

Jill, 27: "Crazy," "loony tunes," "nuts," "off their rocker."

Aileen, 54: They don't particularly bother me.

Black Madonna, 36: Crazy – I hate the word crazy.

Christen, 44: I don't like people calling me "crazy" or "stupid."

Brian, 43: I don't use any terms for the illness, but I sometimes jokingly refer to the hospital as "the funny farm" or the "loony bin."

Jay, 56: Disease.

Liana, 50: Someone just reminded me, they said, "You're talking through your hat."

Have you ever felt that others thought you were inferior to them because of your mental illness? What would you say to these people?

Jade, 43: It could happen to you!

Socrates, 43: One of my housemates "talks down" to me, and I feel like one of my coworkers does as well. A lot of people don't realize that some of the mentally ill are actually quite intelligent. I would encourage people to treat the mentally ill with dignity and respect.

Brunhilda, 44: Most of my delusions are centered around others criticizing me and my inferiority to them. Somehow this seems to mimic real life. I would tell these people, "Life is about that you like, not what you hate."

Will, 38: Yes, they'll learn, eventually. I know and like myself for what I am. If they cannot embrace that, they are the ones who have lost, not I.

> In the middle ages, the term for people with mental illness was "lunatics" stemming from the term "lunacy" which means influenced by the moon. They were deemed witches and were thought to be possessed by evil spirits (Lunatic 6).

Jane, 53: I am not sure that people have treated me as inferior because of my illness, but I think my relatives have treated me as if I were different than they were, and perhaps as if they were not always certain what I was going to understand and what I wouldn't. I don't have any special message to them, but I think of them with love.

Barnaby, 23: I have been in that situation. I don't know if I'd say anything; they're probably not worth it. It does make me mad, though.

Harriet, 43: Yes. "I'll prove you wrong."

Larry, 46: Yes, I would hope they would look at me for who I am today and continue to help me in my struggle to lead a full life.

Jill, 27: Yes, and I would say, "mental illness is a brain disorder, not a disgrace."

Black Madonna, 36: Yes, that mental illness is a brain disease, and just as AIDS or cancer or diabetes is a medical illness, mental illness should be labeled as the same.

Brian, 43: Yes, and I would say to these people that they must have a pretty small mind or they would not think that way. I would also say to them that I am equal to them in every way and that I am the same as any other human being.

Jay, 56: Yes – nothing. Withdraw.

Liana, 50: A friend that I knew from high school said, "You get your words mixed up." I thought, "Well, maybe that's not entirely true."

Do you think others are afraid of you because of your mental illness? What would you like to say to those people?

Jade, 43: Just get to know me—you'll see there's nothing to fear.

Socrates, 43: When my coworker first learned, she was a little fearful; but now she loves me, because I've shown her there's nothing to fear. I think if people were more tolerant of "deviations from the norm," this would be a better place.

Danny Green, 46: Yes – Beware!

Brunhilda, 44: I had a neighbor who tried taking advantage of me repeatedly. She hated the system so I recommended a funny book called *Getting Even*. She was taken aback by the title (didn't even read it). She now thinks I'm not nice like she originally thought—just a dangerous crazy. Now she leaves me alone. Works for me.

Will, 38: Nothing. They're probably wasting time in situations that are less satisfying and more oppressive just to feel "safe."

A movement has begun, called the Campaign to Abolish the Schizophrenia Label, to reduce the stigma of schizophrenia by changing the name. A prominent supporter of the CASL suggests that the term is associated with "violence, dangerousness, unpredictability, inability to recover and constant illness" (Mental 4).

Jane, 53: One person seemed afraid that I would engage in hostile behavior against her, and I am very sorry for that. I would like to tell her that I have not had that kind of feeling or even a wild thought of that for a long time, and that I certainly did not have such a thought toward her!

Barnaby, 23: I had one friend, a good friend, that I lost because of his presuppositions. He never tried to understand—he just avoided me. I was actually supposed to room with him in the dorm at college, but when I started to get sick, he stopped being my friend. I feel like he stabbed me in the back. I don't have anything to say to him. I don't care so much any more.

Larry, 46: No, I would say it's all right to be hesitant, but don't completely undermine the stereotype.

Jill, 27: Sometimes, "Do I not look human?—if you prick me do I not bleed?" etc.

Black Madonna, 36: Yes, because of the stigma, and the way some people stereotype people who kill others who have mental illness – or maybe because of the violence that is associated with mental illness.

Christen, 44: I would say to those people, "Don't be afraid of me as long as I take my medicine."

Brian, 43: I think that "Joe Public" is probably pretty afraid of people who have mental illness because of what has been pounded into their minds by the media, and I would just say to them not to believe everything they hear on the TV or in the newspaper.

Liana, 50: Sometimes I think little children are disgusted about my drug dependency. I would like to say, "I don't blame you one bit!"

Elaborations...

Jade, 43: I went to buy this antique mirror in Alamance County, and a woman asked me what I did for a living. I stumbled a little bit, and then said, "I work at Club Nova Thrift Shop."

She said, "Oh, that's wonderful! I like to shop there. They give the money to take care of the mentals."

I almost broke up laughing, but I contained myself until I was out of the store and could share the story with my dad.

Brunhilda, 44: When I went on the antipsychotic Clozaril, approximately 15 years ago, I found that it caused me to have a disorder of attention. Previously, I had been through stages where I was quite a bookworm. There were periods where I lived in my own world of books, avidly staying up all night to finish a book. Today I have to try hard just to finish my morning paper, *Newsweek*, and short articles in numerous magazines.

Five years ago, I decided to enter some artwork in *Brushes with Life: Art, Artists and Mental Illness*, currently a biannual exhibit at the hospital and several traveling exhibits a year. (Included were exhibits at the North Carolina Museum of Art, RDU airport, a community college, a coffee shop and a restaurant.) In college, I had a beginning oil painting class and I hated it. So I decided I would try acrylic painting. I discovered I could paint for hours, without losing concentration or becoming frustrated. When I started, I wasn't very good. *Brushes with Life* was so motivating because the worst thing people will say about your art work is that it's "nice." Even the better paintings are "nice." There is no pressure on me when I paint, as opposed to other art forms that I'm better at.

My first entry in *Brushes with Life* was five multi-media abstracts. I took the NAMI logo and embellished the abstract representing the brain. In one, I used crumpled paper, one I put in a box, one brain was represented by yarn in knots, and another one was represented by a silver screw. On the large logo, I glued pills, titling it "Pillhead." I think most people with mental illness can relate to some or all of these analogies. I even asked my resident: "What would you do if you had a patient who depicts their brain as a big screw?" He did!

Brian, 43: I feel very strongly that mental illnesses are biological brain disorders and are no one's fault. Not even our parents. Also, I reject all stigma and prejudice regarding mental illness and the people who suffer from it.

On the issue of stigma I think that people with mental illness should not feel that they have to hide their illness or feel ashamed of themselves because of their illness. I feel that we have nothing at all to be ashamed of, and I feel that people who have mental illness all over the country should have a "coming out" the same way gay people have done, which has brought such a positive change all over the world. I think that a "coming out" of people with mental illness all over the country would serve to dispel the myths of mental illness and would help a great deal in erasing the stigma which is so prevalent in our society. This stigma is as bad as racism and as ignorant as homophobia and is equally as damaging to people who have the illness and their families. And I think that a positive, proactive approach such as this would be as effective in fighting the bigotry surrounding mental illness as it has been for the civil rights movement or the gay rights movement.

Our Voices:
Concluding Comments from
the Author-Editors

Your Brain is All in Your Head

By Pickens Miller

Imagine walking into your nephrologist's office and being told you had a bad kidney. Would you feel insulted? Would you expect to be distrusted and blamed and punished for your own renal failure? Now suppose you walked into your dermatologist's office with a rash that was quite apparent to you both. Is it shingles? Psoriasis? Does the doctor have the expertise to make the proper diagnosis? In either case, you probably would not take the evaluation personally or that it represented a shortcoming on your part. Furthermore, you could be certain, especially with second and third opinions, that the diagnosis was either on target or it missed the mark.

Brains, kidneys, and skin are all tissues that form the human body. And the preposterous lie that there is some holy barrier between the physical and the mental, between the body and the mind, has hampered psychiatry and psychology to this day. This false dichotomy is highly dangerous. What could be more physical than the central nervous system? Today neurology and neurobiology are eradicating this distinction.

Schizophrenia is something either you have or you don't. It is a rash you cannot see, just as kidney failure you cannot see. But there *are* symptoms. Are there ever! Because the diagnosis is still somewhat mysterious and scary to the layperson, and because it happens to only one percent of the world's population, people tend to write it off and even ridicule the notion of schizophrenia, as when they engage in gallows humor about death. There are as many synonyms and phrases (most of them derogatory) for "crazy" as there are for "drunk."

Blindness is perhaps the easiest disability to visualize. All one needs to do is to shut one's eyes or deploy a blindfold for a day. A person whose legs no longer work can be understood to have challenging days that persist day after day. Can you also perceive a complete dysfunction of one's brain?

Only now have we developed medicines that can combat schizophrenia. Millions of people worldwide finally have some hope for healing. Seventy-five million of us in all countries, societies, and cultures could begin to approximate life with relief from the disease's oppressive and sometimes deadly symptoms if we had access to these medications. Psychiatry itself suffers a poor reputation among many sectors of society. This is not entirely undeserved. The stereotypes of psychiatric treatment involving lobotomies, electric shock therapy, couches, snakepits, strait jackets, excruciating tranquilizers, four-point restraints, pee-soaked mattresses in "quiet rooms," (not to mention the bizarre note pads, Rorschach tests, "multi-phasic" tests, dream interpretation) all lend ammunition to a huge skepticism towards the psychiatric profession. And when you add the "men in white suits," rubber rooms, and an obscenely observational approach towards its patients, then you begin to get the picture.

There are still lay people who associate schizophrenia with criminality possibly because every single murderer seems to claim insanity as a defense. Yet, of the many people I know with mental illness, we never use our diagnosis to excuse ourselves of anything. We take full responsibility for all our own actions.

Schizophrenia is as physical as kidney failure and as real as a rash. In its severest form, it produces a complete shutdown of all the brain's functions of intellect and emotion. Clinical depression involves dread and the annihilation of will. Schizophrenia causes outright terror and the annihilation of purpose. Naturally, the resulting isolation and confusion trouble both the sufferer and all those around him. The channels of communication get scrambled and strained. If the sufferer cannot articulate the damage, just think how terribly hard it is for the sufferer's family. In schizophrenia, you cannot think, you cannot feel, and you cannot explain.

Sometimes we seek an avenue in religion to explain our experiences and to help us feel. And yet psychiatry bristles with hostility toward religion. The only reason that the stories behind Abraham, Job, Jesus, and Allah resonate so powerfully with schizoaffective, affective, and schizophrenic sufferers is simply that there exist no other metaphors big enough to fit the pain and confusion brought on by these diseases. In many psychiatric wards the staff labor to ward off what they insist are "false beliefs." I'm not sure that there are any religions out there that don't put a considerable strain on one's rational powers.

In my experience, there is another side of psychiatry worth mentioning. This is along the tilting axis of being told (on the one hand) that I was a horrible danger and that something is decidedly wrong with me, and then being told (on the other hand) that I am a malingerer and that nothing is wrong with me at all. And both these accusations were made by the exact same people, in alternate harmony.

People frequently use our diagnosis both to deligitimize our own perspective on events, and also to justify their violence against us. Because they feel they can abuse us with no fear of consequence, and often with complete impunity, they believe that by undercutting our credibility in the case of a perceived threat that they can get away with all violence towards us, including murder. Their mantra is always that "they are worried" about us, and then proceed to attack us or, in a punitive fit with no reasonable alibi, place us in a hospital to hide their own culpability.

Of course, in a medical crisis, we belong in the hospital. If the reasons are therapeutic and not punitive, the hospital represents a welcome respite, refuge, and asylum where our scientific advancements in developing the exactly right medicines may be put to good use. And as for the care-givers: no Nazis need apply! If you have a brown-shirted mindset, please find another line of work. In all my time with the "care-givers," I've always felt far more threatened by the staff than by the same patients who are purportedly "a danger to themselves or others."

When locked within wards, I was treated worse and with less re-spect than the gazelles on "Wild Kingdom." In the 1970s and early 80s, I was inundated with harmful, damaging, and toxic drugs. I have never felt worse than when under their influence. For those in locked psych wards, with none of the legal restraints in place governing most jails and prisons, and often with no access to an attorney, wardens may treat their patients indifferently, or well, or with criminal malice, from one hospital to another. Toxic "medicines" and "quiet" rooms are two technically non-criminal controlling techniques of preference in many hospitals. Most of the time, however, these short-sighted tactics are chosen for short-term behavior management and not for therapeutic strategies for the long term.

With deinstitutionalization beginning in the 1950s until this very moment, has come under-employment, unemployment, homelessness, hunger, lack of access to medicine, and total isolation and despair.

What society gains in the short term by ignoring the medical needs of its citizens who face schizophrenia and schizoaffective disease, it los-es far more by every measurement in the long term. There was a time in the United States when we were even denied suffrage. Although we've always paid our own payroll taxes and our own income taxes, and although the first vote I cast was for my father for the U.S. Senate, the powers that be still treat us like outcasts. Sometimes I feel enfranchised, and sometimes I feel estranged in my own country. I worked for 30 years while fighting my schizophrenia, and even that was dismissed as inadequate. Perhaps not so strangely there exists a nearly perfect cor-relation between schizophrenia and lifelong poverty.

While it's hard enough to be perpetually employed and always in non-skilled jobs, my education was predictably truncated by the onset of my diagnosis, and for many this happens in midstream or even ear-lier in our academic careers. With extreme courage, many of my friends have gone back to secondary schools, college and graduate schools. Without this courage, we would not get to return to jobs that require highly skilled applicants. And without at least a high school diploma, many of us would not be able to re-enter the workforce at all. We certainly want to earn our own livings. My own life has had me mainly filling one unskilled job after another for 30 years. My schooling ended at age 15, and I only earned my high school diploma while living in a psych ward with the help of public school tutors.

Because no one is to blame for schizophrenia, we need to stop putting parents, siblings and sufferers at fault. There is nothing to be gained and a great deal of damage to be done by assigning responsibility for what is a strictly biochemical deficit. Whether genetic or not, and most evidence points in the genetic direction, the remedies for mental illness all seem to be medical. This was not true in the 1970s. Now there is hope!

I've always said "If we walk off into the sunset with the utmost haste, the sun shall never set." Since none of us can walk that fast, one century from now (and two, three, four), there will be whole new generations of people facing schizophrenia and schizoaffective disorder. The upshot of this crisis shall surely incorporate the best medicines of today with even better ones yet to be developed. Public ignorance and fear may wither and fade away.

In the late 18th century when King George III of England exhibited strange behavior and suffered from what his doctors called "madness," there was a great surge in British public opinion that, if the King could come down with mental illness, then anyone could. Attitudes shifted. People hoped that from then on, psychiatric troubles would be addressed on a par with other maladies.

Of course, that never happened. As every amateur historian knows, King George's madness began when his liver failed him. This liver condition, porphyria, can still cause mental illness. Even English cattle can go mad. Brain diseases are by no means restricted to our own species.

Here is my wish list for the upcoming centuries:

1. Diseases of the brain shall all be treated with absolute urgency. No brain tumor or autism or schizophrenia will go unattended. The brain and the lungs and the liver will be on par.
2. Our homelessness will be an ancient, ugly memory. We will all have a home.
3. Advice and consent shall govern all interactions between doctor and patient. And once medicine is prescribed and taken, the patient's own assessment of whether a medicine is working and how effective it is shall be a chief consideration.
4. Physical and other abuse by psychiatric ward staff must stop.
5. There will be strict laws prohibiting the purchase of firearms.
6. All crimes committed against us shall be prosecuted.
7. Unless the primary diagnosis is medical, we'll no longer be lumped together with criminals and drug offenders.

Overall, I dream of a day, as have others before, when we shall share in the American Dream. And the "promissory note" begun under the Americans with Disabilities Act enacted by Congress, sponsored by Kennedy and Domenici, can be deposited in the currency of equal respect among our countrymen. While most of you have had no idea what we've encountered over the centuries, perhaps this book will prime your education.

Addressing Schizophrenia's Four-Pronged Assault

By Michael Dunne

First, I would like to thank Colette for bringing me in on this project. This book was her brainchild, and I have learned a great deal about schizophrenia through the process of forming this book. Colette is a lot more talented than she gives herself credit for, and I hope that her work on this book has shown her that.

There is a lot I could say about mental illness, and I am glad that I have the opportunity to do so briefly now. What is my take on the illness? The first conclusion I have drawn from reading these first-person accounts is that the illness manifests differently in different people. Not only is each of our chemical systems different from one another and thus we react differently to different medications, but also, every person is unique, with different experiences, different responses to these experiences, different viewpoints, and different beliefs. But one thing is universal: schizophrenia is an illness that affects us physically, emotionally, psychologically and spiritually. Therapy must address each of these elements of our being, if real healing is going to take place.

Great strides have taken place on the physical level. For most, the second-generation medications have fewer side effects and allow us to potentially function at high levels. Though finding the best medication for the given individual is often a hit-or-miss process, and thus so many of us have tried a great number of them, I believe that strides will continue to be made on this front. Finding a medication that works for you, one that limits symptoms and doesn't make life unbearable, is the first step to recovery. Sometimes accepting that you will have to be on drugs for the rest of your life is difficult, but once you accept this reality, you have begun to own your illness. Lots of people have to take medication for various conditions for the rest of their lives; taking medication is nothing to be ashamed of. Thank God and man that we have these new drugs to allow us to cope; many in the past did not.

Mental illness also affects us emotionally. Everyone has emotional baggage, none of us skate through life without emotional scars, and often those that develop mental illness have many. Professionals can help us identify these scars and direct us how to respond to them in ways that will help heal us. The illness itself adds to any pre-existing scars, because developing mental illness is a kind of emotional death. You may lose part of yourself: coping ability, cognitive ability, education, employment, family and friends. Most people do not understand the illness, and you may feel alone with your illness, but I think this book shows that you are not alone. Sure there is stigma, which results from ignorance, but once you own your illness and accept yourself, you can transcend others' misguided judgments and develop new self-esteem. Of course, healing on the physical level helps with this work.

The psychological aspect of the illness is affected by the physical and incorporates the emotional, but it goes beyond these two elements. We must learn to think differently. This work can be difficult and painful, and healing emotionally aids it, but basically, you must learn to identify destructive thinking patterns and substitute new patterns. You must learn when you have negative self-perceptions and correct them to bolster your self-esteem. You must learn not to worry about what others may be thinking about you and not fear their judgments. Doing so will cut down on paranoia and delusions. When you hear a negative voice, ignore it if you can. Think positively of others, and you may be amazed at how they respond to you. None of these things are easy to do, but doing so will improve your heart and mind. Mental health professionals can help you with this work, and know that not just people with mental illness need to correct their way of thinking.

This psychological work borders on spirituality. Because how we treat, respond and interact with others is part of all spiritual frameworks. And it is this element of mental illness that is largely ignored because it's often misunderstood and therefore feared. Professionals may not share your belief system, since our beliefs are based on our experiences, and no two people have exactly the same experiences. And how we respond to them may differ, but it has been my experience that there is definitely a spiritual aspect to this illness. The spiritual element involves the unseen dimension, and therefore can only be believed, not proven. You can't prove the existence of a spiritual realm to another, but many would agree that it still exists. Often we *feel* people looking at us, because their spirits flow from their being and touch us in some way. I would stipulate that many with schizophrenia feel the unseen dimension more acutely than "normal" people. Many with mental illness feel like somehow they are being invaded. And just like someone cannot prove that voices are only your brain backfiring on itself, I cannot prove that they are malicious spirits harassing us. But if you had lived in my body for the last 18 years and had my experiences, you would have no doubt that that is what they are.

So how do you deal with the spiritual aspect of the illness if your doctor and social worker think it's a manifestation of your illness? What has worked for me is meditation and prayer. Whatever your faith is, I would encourage you to use it to address your illness. If you believe in God or a Higher Power, try to focus on this entity within yourself. Even professionals would agree that meditation helps focus and can give peace. Spend a half-hour a day doing this, and you may be surprised at what happens. When I feel afflicted, I start meditating and it results in not only a psychological response, but also a physical one. And once my being is released, peace returns to me and I am back to my baseline.

So, I would encourage all those with mental illness and those close to them to have hope. When things are bad and you're in a dark tunnel, it is hard to have hope, but that is the essence of faith. Strides are being made in understanding and responding to this devastating illness, and though you may never return to how you were before your illness, the process of looking within can yield growth. You may have to come to know yourself in a new way, but it is possible, though not easy, to emerge from the darkness a changed person, one that understands his or her shortcomings and strengths, and accepts himself or herself and those around them with more kindness and humility.

The Power of the Mind to Heal

By Claudia Moon

My life was out of control. I hung myself in a hospital. I was determined to end my life. My voices were commanding me to do so. Some staff members judged me. They said I had anger issues. I was seeing dead bodies and hearing voices and they were telling me to write positive remarks in a journal. One psychiatrist at the fancy plush hospital told me I was not living up to hospital etiquette. I didn't know up from down; I was so psychotic her lips were turning blue in front of me; I thought she was dead and I had killed her. My voices told me to run away as fast as I could.

It wasn't until a doctor diagnosed me with schizoaffective disorder that I began to get the treatment I needed. She recognized that I was really sick, and she began medicating me properly. I trusted her and took the medication.

Even with the medication, I was chronically psychotic for almost 10 years, in hospitals for a total of five years and many months.

My outside time was hell. People I trusted encouraged me to live in a nursing home. My fiercely independent nature knew that would never happen. Until recently I was adamant about my independent living arrangement. Now I have a husband, and we balance our time together with alone time. We need both for our hearts and minds to heal and grow.

I guess what I've learned in the last 10 years is never underestimate the power for the mind to heal.

People who judged me along the way could never help me because I was sensitive to their judgments; they had made up their minds about me, leaving me no room to grow. People who supported me along the way have a special place in my heart. It was their faith that in the depths of my soul and heart was something worth saving. And, even in my deepest psychotic stages, I was able to trust and connect with them. That core connection, along with exercise, my faith, and my relationships, has brought me closer to healing.

Things Are Looking Up

By Manisha Kapil

We have reasons for optimism for the treatment of mental illness in the U.S. With the advent of expensive atypical antipsychotic medications on the market and other societal measures, I believe that the way that the larger world copes with those who have brain disease will ease and get better.

In the chapter on finance, you can read how closely mental illness and poverty are tied. The role of economic factors is increasingly important for people with mental illness, as the price of medications and needed treatments continue to play a role in their recovery. It could be argued that there is so much pressure to see results in the treatment of brain disorders that the cost to the consumer is irrelevant. We however, struggle with Abilify being $ 14.00 a pill! (Thank Goodness for Medicaid!)

In North Carolina I am concerned about the demise of the state psychiatric hospital. State psychiatric hospitals were a refuge for the severely ill. As they close, the persons with brain disorders are released to community care, on to the streets.

One answer has been to develop assertive community treatment (ACT) teams, that call for a team of professionals, on call to patients and families 24 hours a day, every day of the year. They provide psychiatric treatment, therapy, case management, community-based support, and outreach.

Only a handful of states (North Carolina, Delaware, Idaho, Michigan, Rhode Island, Texas, and Wisconsin) currently have statewide ACT programs (also called PACT). Nineteen states and the District of Columbia have at least one or more pilot programs in their state.

In addition to assertive and community-based services, one positive change has been jail diversion programs. These, like the Community Resources Court in Chapel Hill, provide the community with treatment-based options to incarceration. Which is a good thing.

You see, since the State Psychiatric Hospital is a diminishing concept, the severely ill have a tendency to act out their "problem," which can involve law enforcement and possible jail time.

What I conclude from the book is that the problems we have as schizophrenics are manifold. Other than the issues we have with the law, we have problems in our personal lives. Because of the issues discussed above, we face problems with interpersonal relationships, such as the question of dating.

We still have personal needs such as the need for companionship and intimacy. How and when do you tell your companion that you have a chronic condition? How and when do you tell your companion that you are taking expensive medication and can't move? There are other questions, but they are best kept inside. Will he care?

Thank goodness for the expensive antipsychotics. They make rational conversations possible.

Basically, thing are looking up.

What You Can Do Now!

By Colette Corr

The mental health care system in the United States is frequently described to be "in crisis" or a "disaster." Looking backwards from the present to 30 years ago, experts have always used these same terms when describing inadequate government policies and legislation, lack of funding for treatment, research and essential programs for the mentally ill. Changing the system is a slow process and sometimes it appears to be "trial and error," always seeking "what works," in the best manner possible. Mental health reform is necessary at all levels—local, state and federal. What can you do now? Become an advocate; lobby for important legislation, fight stigma, and above all, VOTE!

Join private organizations that can help you advocate, educate and combat stigma. Fighting stigma creates the ability to make legislative changes. By altering public opinion and furthering the understanding of severe mental illness (including schizophrenia), we gain support for important bills and funding. These nonprofit organizations monitor primarily the news and entertainment industries. The National Alliance for the Mentally Ill (NAMI) at www.nami.org offers "stigma alerts" and helps show you how and with whom to take action. "Stigmabusters" allows members to report infractions against people with mental illness, physical as well as verbal. There are other agencies, such as the Carter Center, whose primary goal is to combat the stigma of mental illness. Some of the solutions and goals of these organizations range from national advertisements, distribution and information, education in schools to simply explaining mental illness to your children.

Families with a member who has severe mental illness are the usual spokespeople. E. Fuller Torrey, in *Surviving Schizophrenia*, points out that advocacy from patients themselves adds credibility to the causes, especially when giving feedback about what services are effective and how to improve them. His other three principles to advocacy are: relying on what is factual and not emotional, putting everything in writing (letters, email), meeting with officials, sending copies to all concerned. Also, judging public officials by their actions, not by what they promise.

There is one principal E. Fuller Torrey didn't list: become an expert. Educate, read and research. You may wish to focus on only one area of specialty or adopt a sound opinion from a real expert in one of the pertaining fields.

How do I go about it? Where to start? It's easier than you think, and you don't need to spend that much time. Most activity in mental health reform occurs at the state level. The Treatment Advocacy Center (TAC), a non-profit organization, has a detailed website of databases that contain all laws pertaining to mental illness and are searchable by state. A detailed and extensive website, TAC gives comments on public policy, news and alerts. They monitor what is printed and notify you when legislation in your state will be voted on. You can look up who is representing you by zip code as well as the current legislative calendar.

NAMI also has website for all three levels—national, state and local. Go to the homepage at www.nami.org and click on "action." They have national legislative alerts and updates, and a section called "Megavote" that monitors how your Representative or Senator votes. They have tips on writing letters and making phone calls to your representatives. You can even email your legislators from this website. You can't get it any easier than that.

The North Carolina NAMI (www.naminc.org) even has the entire expose series of articles written and researched by the *News and Observer* in Raleigh. These articles triggered the "reform of the Mental Health system 2000." This is an exciting period in mental health advocacy in North Carolina, after much scandal. The NAMI state-level website has current legislative issues and news alerts as well.

The local individual NAMI websites vary—some are impressive, some are less than adequate for advocacy. I would suggest you consult a social worker at your local state hospital or mental health facility. Perhaps they can add you to an organized list of people alerted and notified by email when local advocacy is needed. It doesn't take long to write a short email and send it to everyone on a list provided for you.

Log on to NCMentalHealthVote.org or a similar website for your state. Vote for who you believe is right!

Vote because together we are strong.

Above all, just vote!

The Our Voices Book Committee

The committee of authors for this project are five men and women who each manage a mental illness of schizophrenia or schizoaffective disorder. They live, work, make friends, and contribute to communities in central North Carolina. They all have in common a small clinic in Chapel Hill, where they also met two clinical social workers and invited them to join in this journey.

Colette Corr
Colette has battled schizoaffective disorder for 26 years. After experiencing chronic psychosis for several years, she graduated from Meredith College in Raleigh, NC. After a series of failed employments at various levels, she went on disability 10 years after the onset of her mental illness. Later, she retrained by obtaining an AAS in horticulture and at the time was designated the hardest worker at her workplace. She has many hobbies, including gardening and painting.

Mike Dunne
Mike was diagnosed with schizoaffective disorder in 1989. He has a BA in English and an MA in Teaching English from UNC-Chapel Hill and has worked (among other occupations) as a roadie, private investigator, laborer and teacher. He currently manages a bookstore and is writing his first novel. He has published several poems in anthologies and hopes one day to publish a poetry collection.

Manisha Kapil
Manisha graduated from the University of Wisconsin in 1983, with a Bachelors degree in French Language and Literature and from the City Colleges of Chicago, with an Advanced Certificate in Travel and Tourism in 1989. Originally from Wisconsin, she currently resides in Raleigh where she has been for the last 10 years. She has resided in Paris, France and Ankara, Turkey. Manisha was diagnosed with a chronic condition five years ago and is under treatment at UNC-Chapel Hill.

Claudia Moon

Claudia is an avid reader, swimmer and poet. She follows legislation affecting people with mental illness and communicates the news in her clubhouse newsletter. She loves music and is usually plugged in. She has and enjoys many friendships and family relationships. She hopes to see a brighter future for those living with mental illness.

Pickens Miller

Pickens first noticed the symptoms of schizoaffective disorder at age 15 and was diagnosed at age 17. When not in the hospital, he worked for the next 30 years, but is now on the "D.L."—the disabled list. For the first 21 years of his working life, he was not on any form of disability assistance. After his third suicide attempt at age 38, he qualified for assistance and still worked for another seven years.

Jenny Edwards and Bebe Smith

Jenny and Bebe are two clinical social workers in the Schizophrenia Treatment and Evaluation Program (STEP) Clinic of the University of North Carolina's Department of Psychiatry.

Works Cited

Books, Periodicals, and Newspapers

Anderson, Stephen B. "All About John Beard." *Reintegration Today* Sept.- Nov. 2005: 12-15.

Carmichael, Mary. "Stronger, Faster, Smarter." *Newsweek* 26 Mar. 2007: 38-46

"College Life: Fun & Excitement or Anxiety & Stress?" *Reintegration Today* Sept.-Nov. 2005: 16-18.

Drummond, Mike. "Lack of Arms Doesn't Stop Her." *News and Record* [Greensboro] 28 Dec. 2007: B4B.

Duckworth, Ken. "Diabetes: Winning the Battle." *NAMI Advocate* June- Aug. 2007: 4-7.

"From Lunatic to Consumer". *Reintegration Today* Dec.-Feb. 2008: 6-7.

"Mental Health Experts Debate Use of the Term 'Schizophrenia.'" *Reintegration Today* Dec.-Feb. 2008: 4.

Miller, Rachel and Susan E. Mason. *Diagnosis Schizophrenia: A Comprehensive Resource for Patients, Families, and Helping Professionals.* New York: Columbia UP, 2002.

Miller, Michael Craig. "Exercise is a State of Mind." *Newsweek* 26 Mar. 2007: 48-55.

Mueser, Kim D., and Susan Gingerich. *Coping with Schizophrenia: A Guide for Families*. Oakland, CA: New Harbinger, 1994.

Noll, Richard. *The Encyclopedia of Schizophrenia and Other Psychotic Disorders*. 3rd ed. New York: Facts on File, 2007.

Smith, Barbara, ed. *A Family Guide to Severe Mental Illness*. Chapel Hill, NC: UNC STEP and MHA Orange County, 2003.

Torrey, E. Fuller. *Surviving Schizophrenia: A Manual for Families, Patients and Providers*. 5th ed. New York: Collins, 2006.

"The Uninsured and Costs of Mental Illness." *NAMI Advocate* June-Aug 2007: 8-11.

Web Sites

www.ajp.psychiatryonline.org   www.psychiatry.unc.edu

www.census.gov   www.schizophrenia.com

www.mentalhealth.samhsa.gov   www.who.int

www.psychlaws.org   www.wikipedia.org

•••••••••

Printed in the United States
133461LV00002B/121-312/P

9 781440 110399